Contents

Sotai
Natural Exercise

by Keizo Hashimoto, M. D.
translated by Herman Aihara

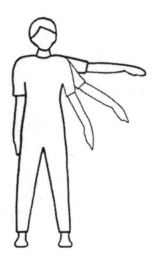

George Ohsawa Macrobiotic Foundation
Chico, California

Other Books by Herman Aihara
Acid and Alkaline
Basic Macrobiotics
Kaleidoscope
Learning from Salmon
Macrobiotics: An Invitation to Health and Happiness
Milk, A Myth of Civilization
Natural Healing from Head to Toe

Cover design by Carl Campbell
Text layout and design by Carl Ferré

First published in Japanese	1977
First English Edition	1981
Current Printing: edited and reformatted	2010 Aug 25

Published with the help of East West Center for Macrobiotics
www.eastwestmacrobiotics.com

ISBN 978-0-918860-33-0

Foreword

The first thing you have to understand before you learn this sotai exercise is that Nature designed and built us in such a way that we can live our whole life healthfully and happily. However, we often live against this natural design and make ourselves sick and unhappy; if we make ourselves sick and unhappy, then we simply must return our body to its natural condition.

Sotai is the exercise that brings our body back to the natural condition. It is not the normal kind of exercise intended to build muscles such as athletic or training exercises.

When most people do not feel well, they go to doctors who take X-rays, examine blood pressure, heartbeat, and even brain waves with expensive machinery. Furthermore, they check the urine, blood, and other body fluids chemically. After gathering the data from all the tests, the doctors decide what kind of sicknesses the patient is suffering from. The patient is released from worry about his suffering when he is given a fancy name for the sickness—such as atherosclerosis, diabetes, etc.

However, curing the sickness is not so smooth. Furthermore, there are many cases in which doctors cannot give any specific name for the sufferings claimed by the patients. In such cases, doctors don't know how to treat patients.

Because I became a medical doctor fifty years ago, I have had many cases in which I couldn't give specific names for the symptoms, not to mention the treatment. Recently I reached the idea by which I can explain the cause of those sicknesses and treat them successfully. This book is the result of my fifty-year practice of medicine. By this, you can correct your suffering that medical doctors often cannot.

In order to publish this book, I am indebted to Dr. Yukinori Hashimoto of *Modern Agriculture* magazine, who inspired me to publish my work. I must also give my greatest appreciation to the publisher of this book (the director of the Farmer's and Fisherman's Cultural Association) and Mr. M. Shigenuki, who has been supporting my ideas.

– Keizo Hashimoto, M.D.

Foreword to the English Edition

Why does man have to suffer from sicknesses? Nature (God) planned man perfectly so that he can live in good health. Western medicine developed based on a pathological, anatomical, and histological concept of medicine. Oriental medicine realized that one of the causes of sickness is deformation or imbalance existing in the basic body construction. Oriental medicine succeeded in correcting those deformations or imbalances by the stimulation of acupuncture reflex points. However, it has not yet tried to correct deformations by body motions or movements.

From my fifty years of experience, I reached the firm conclusion that the movement or motion that is in the opposite direction of the pain—in other words, movement that brings a good feeling—will correct bodily deformation or imbalance. However, right motion is not the only condition for healthy living. For this, man must establish the right order and balance in breathing, eating and drinking, body movements, and spiritual activities (thinking, emotion). These activities are all voluntary movements; we can change them by our will. In other words, our health or sickness depends on our choice of these activities. However, most people do not know right breathing, diet, movement, or mental activities.

This book is a guidebook of body movements that will cure many sicknesses and keep people healthy. You cannot believe what I say, but please try some of them. You will find that what I say is right. Health is not a miracle. Health is the state Nature planned for us, and this should be achieved in a comfortable way. If we move our body in the comfortable direction, the body achieves a healthy condition. This is Nature. Please find this out for yourself.

There is one secret in my sotai exercise. Please move the part of the body slowly and easily to the point where comfortable movement of the arm or leg ends, hold that point for a few seconds, and then quickly release all the force. This is the secret of the sotai exercise movement that has cured thousands of sicknesses in Japan.

In the East as well as the West, medical care has been given by others. A few people in olden times knew how to cure sicknesses by themselves, but they left no record. Therefore, the methods of self-curing have been hidden from sight. I fortunately found one of those secrets and have applied it to thousands of people with good results for fifty years. My method has been published in Japan and has benefited thousands; now this book has been translated into English and is going to be published in America.

Because I know sotai will help many suffering people, my happiness is not only selfish but also altruistic. At the same time, I have no way to express my appreciation to Mr. and Mrs. Herman Aihara who painstakingly worked on the translation of my book from Japanese to English.

– Keizo Hashimoto, M.D.
June 1980

Introduction
by Cornellia Aihara

How I Learned Sotai Exercise

When I was in the 6th grade, Japan was at war with China. My teacher chose me and one other person in my class as medical assistants to help the wounded during the war. We bandaged and carried the wounded on stretchers and did many things to help them. I was like a trainee to help wounded men in battle. Two persons from each 6th grade class were chosen to do this.

One day a professional finger massage person came to my school and taught us how to massage all parts of the body. After school, I would go home and tell my parents what I learned that day. I would practice this massage on my father. He was so happy after I massaged him. I would give both my parents a massage from time to time. I remember I used to give my grandmother a shoulder massage, and the next day her shoulders would expand and she had a little pain. So I realized that one should probably change the strength of the massage depending on the age of the person receiving it. I gave a massage that was too strong for my grandmother.

I also thought finger massage should be used on middle-aged or older persons, but after opening Vega Institute it seemed to be the younger generation that needed do-in, yoga, and finger massage. Most of the young people had taken many drugs, so I think their bodies became older than their age.

About seven years ago at the French Meadows Summer Camp, two do-in teachers came from Japan. They came with a group of macrobiotic Japanese touring the United States. After summer camp, I studied do-in with them. While I was in Japan in 1975, I planned to study do-in. I told my mother and sister. My sister is a busy woman, but she sent two letters advising me to study sotai exercise instead of do-in. She recommended sotai because it is simple and effective. So I asked her if I could learn sotai in one month. She recommended Reverend Sakuyama, a disciple of Dr. Keizo Hashimoto. Reverend Sakuyama came to my mother's house in Aizuwakamatsu and taught me several times; I studied with him a total of about one month. He took me to Sendai City and introduced me to Dr. Hashimoto.

I also wanted to study do-in in Kanagawa prefecture, but, unfortunately, the trains were on strike for a long time so I missed my opportunity to study do-in.

In 1977, I returned to Japan and studied sotai with Reverend Sakuyama again. He taught me very well because he said he knew we were running Vega Institute. He chose me to develop sotai exercise in America. He also knew macrobiotic philosophy and diet, and planned to start a similar kind of dojo in Japan. He was Dr. Hashimoto's favorite student.

Dr. Hashimoto was born in the same town as I was. He has been a medical doctor in Sendai City for a long time. He studied macrobiotic philosophy from George Ohsawa. During World War II, he was captured by the Russians and sent to Siberia. They tried to brainwash and convert him to communism. They were not successful in brainwashing him because he understood macrobiotic philosophy. He then appreciated George Ohsawa. When he was a young man, he had much mental suffering; his character was too sensitive. In order to solve the problem, he studied Christianity. He met a good teacher. Since then, he no longer suffers from the sins of man. He found a new world.

I went to Sendai City and met Dr. Hashimoto for the first time. At the time of my visit he was working at his own clinic with about five students. He was a gentle man. He was quiet and did not talk much—like a samurai.

He published a book called *Treatment for Curing all Diseases*. I would like to introduce this book in America because if we study the teachings of this book many Americans will be helped. I recommend sotai exercise because it can be done in 15 minutes. Other exercises of this nature such as do-in, yoga, etc., take a longer time and if you are too busy you won't have enough time to practice them. You will have time to do sotai.

There are two kinds of sotai exercise. One is self-exercise and the other requires an assistant to help you. Practice basic sotai exercises every day for 15 minutes in the morning or evening. Practice basic sotai with helper for an hour once a week or once a month.

When I was in Seattle, there was a man who came to my class; he had been in a car accident and had not been able to sit down for six months. After two or three sotai treatments, he could bend his knees and could also sit down. Sotai exercise balanced his body. We were all surprised to see he could so quickly cure his stiffness caused by the accident. This is the reason I introduced sotai into the United States.

Part 1
Sotai Theory

Why Some Illnesses Cannot Be Cured

Difficult Illnesses

Muscular Dystrophy. A child with muscular dystrophy came to my clinic one day in May of 1975. He could not walk very well, walking on his heels, and he moved shaking his shoulders and hips. He had been abnormal since he was two and is now about 12 years old. He had consulted several doctors in vain. His was the first case of this illness I had ever tried to cure, so I was not sure what to do with him. However, I examined the natural movement of his feet, knees, hips, etc., and I found several deformations. I introduced him to the natural movement exercise (sotai exercise) that is explained in this book. After trying this exercise, he could walk easier and he did not shake his shoulders. His hips did not shake as much as before. His mother was delighted.

Because there are no instruments for examining body conditions in my clinic and this is a very rare disease, I asked my friend's doctor who works in a hospital to take care of him. Knowing my exercise, this doctor gave him a sotai treatment. The boy's CPK (value of blood enzyme) went down from 2000 to 300 (100 is normal value). X-rays showed that his spine had straightened out.

Muscular dystrophy has been considered incurable—one could die from it before reaching 20. However, this boy not only cured this illness but he was now able to swim and could even compete in an athletic meet for the first time in his life.

This case was broadcast on TV. Then several muscular dystrophy patients came to my clinic, and they were improved by sotai exercises. Many doctors are interested in this method now.

Erythema. In 1967, I received a 38-year-old woman as a patient with erythema. She had had an operation to remove her left ovary, her gall bladder, and her left kidney. She had been treated at a university hospital for ten years, but the palms of her hands and the soles of her feet were still red because the skin on those parts was broken. It was difficult for her to walk and to hold objects with her hands. She had pain in her whole body. Her face was the shape of a full moon.

I treated her body deformations with sotai treatment and explained the natural laws of breathing, eating, and mental and physical activity. I asked her to follow this natural law. By eight treatments, the broken skin and redness on the palms of her hands and the soles of her feet were cured. Now she could work harder and more strenuously.

Later, she brought her friend to my clinic. This friend of hers was 27 years old, and she also had the same kind of illness—the palms of her hands and the soles of her feet were red and the skin on those two parts was torn. She wore gloves and wrapped her feet in cotton gauze. She had been treated at a hospital. She came to see me after her second hospitalization. As soon as I gave her sotai treatment, she felt it was easier to breathe. The third time I gave her sotai treatment, her face became smoother. By the fifth time, she became normal.

She had liked sweets extremely. She had eaten pickles with sugar. She had eaten chocolate and 10 quail eggs every day. She had believed that meat and fish are nutritional foods. She did not come for her sixth treatment.

Modern medicine does not know the cause of erythema; therefore modern doctors cannot cure this illness. They can diagnose but cannot cure because they do not know the cause of illness. The cause of illness is in the wrong way of living—breathing, eating, drinking, moving, and thinking. When we correct the wrong way of living, illness is cured naturally.

One of these ways of living is the movement of the body. When our body is deformed, we correct this deformity unconsciously. This is done by instinct. Therefore, we are often cured from illness without any medication. This is the natural healing of our body. However, we can do this natural healing consciously by following the laws of natural movement. This is the sotai exercise I have written about here.

The Shortcomings of Modern Medicine

Modern medicine gave up in curing many illnesses. There was a professional baseball player named Nakanishi. He was a great baseball hitter about 17 years ago. However, he suffered severe pain in his left hand joints. He could not swing the bat. He went to a big university hospital in Japan. The doctors at this hospital could not cure his illness, so he finally went to consult a chiropractor who cured his pain by simply pushing his joint back.

The joints in our hands move by swinging back and forth, going back to normal position by reversing the motion of swing. However, if the hand does not go back to the right position, there remains a deformity and this can cause pain. The chiropractor put the joint back in the right position, which the orthodox hospital could not. There are many such cases.

If you have pain in the hip and go to a doctor, he will take an X-ray first. If he cannot find anything wrong in the bone, he will examine it with some other test. If none of the tests show anything wrong, then he will say "You are tired. Take a rest." If he finds something wrong in the bone, he may say, "The hip bone is out of line." But there is no easy cure for this, because modern medicine does not know what causes it—or anything else for that matter. Modern medicine does not know the cause of disease, but medicines are given at random; that is, modern doctors randomly give out drugs. If the patient is lucky, the medicine the doctor prescribes might cure his illness; if it does not, then the doctor tries some other drug or medicine.

Neuralgia is a good example. The cause of this disease may be an infection in the central nervous system or the peripheral nervous system. However, sometimes the nerve has nothing wrong with it, but the physical force is causing it to feel painful. In such cases, the removal of the physical force is the cure. Modern medicine often overlooks the existence of such physical forces.

What is lacking in modern medicine? I am a medical doctor. The job of a medical doctor is to cure sicknesses. However, modern medicine has not succeeded in curing, in most cases. I think modern medicine has misunderstood sickness. For example, modern medicine developed pathology, which well explains all conditions of diseases. However, patients do not want such an explanation—they just want relief from the suffering and pain of the disease, and prolongation of life. Modern medicine is not successful in this.

Modern medicine developed surgery, which removes both the diseased organ and joint from a person's body. However, this is not the real cure—and the organs are gone forever. Such cases are the removal of tonsils, appendix, ovary, etc. Are these organs really unnecessary? Is surgery really curing disease? I question this tendency of medicine.

In short, modern medicine lacks the study about the human body, which covers the organs and the nervous system. However, most Oriental methods such as moxa, acupuncture, shiatsu massage, and chiropractic treatment are healing from outside the body, not inside. When the internal organs are bad, the external body becomes sick too. In this case, curing the internal organs also cures the outer body. If a person's body is not healthy, then the internal organs are not healthy either; curing the body also cures the internal organs. In this case, modern medicine cannot help, but Oriental medicine does better.

Modern medicine has developed many branches, and specialists are studying in each of these branches. However, there is not much benefit. Now there is a movement to coordinate these specialists. In other words, the specialists will study together toward a conclusion. However, they lack one thing: there is no study of body mechanism as a whole. There are body studies such as physiology and anatomy. However, they study bones and muscles statically and lack study of movement and its potential.

Modern science developed studies such as anatomy, muscle structure, constitution, connection to bones, causes of tiredness (an accumulation of lactic acid), chemical reactions in the stomach, etc. However, they do not relate such knowledge to the whole body. Gathering parts does not make a totality. Curing parts without understanding the whole will be temporal. Medicine must consider the human body as a whole, not an accumulation of parts.

Modern medicine is analytical—analyzing the blood, urine, measuring blood pressure. Then it names the disease. The name gives the way of treatment. However, many modern diseases cannot be diagnosed as disorders of bodily function by such analysis. For example, cancer will not show any signs of the illness by chemical analysis for many years. In such cases, modern medicine has no way to treat the illness.

I admire chemical analysis. It is very important. The most important contribution of chemical analysis is the development in the studies of bacteriology and immunology. This development reduced the rate of infectious diseases. However, this is not the solution for all diseases.

For example, 20 people may eat poisonous foods but not necessarily all will become ill. Eighteen of the people may become ill but two may not become ill. The common cold is a good example. While many become ill from infectious cold, some may not suffer at all. For example, in the case of pollution sickness not all people in an area become sick. Therefore, the chemical is not the only cause of the sickness. Physical body conditions may be the cause too. It is important to study the chemical conditions of the body. However, it is also important to study the physical conditions of the body.

Life is movement. Movement is based on the law of mechanics. Therefore, without the study of the law of mechanics—physical study—modern medicine cannot understand the causes of disease. Here is an important shortcoming of modern medicine.

In order to examine the physical condition of the body, you simply move the body. You will find the easier side and the more difficult side. Then think why one side is more difficult to move. There must be some stress or strain or deformation on that side. This difficulty is related not only to muscles but also to the internal organs.

Modern medicine diagnoses by chemical analysis, and its diagnostics are based on statistics. There are standard values of red blood cells, white blood cells, amount of sugar, protein, etc., in the blood. This is the scale of health or sickness. Here is a problem. Those statistics are not absolute, but average. You may not belong to this value. You may be healthy even though your certain value is not the average value.

For example, someone has a blood pressure of 200. A doctor administers a drug to reduce the blood pressure. However, the patient may have been in better condition when the blood pressure was 200, rather than a lower value. He must be certain of his condition in which a balanced condition was maintained by the blood pressure of 200. When he reduced the blood pressure, he may have created an imbalance just by changing only the blood pressure. By statistics, normal blood pressure is 140/80. If over 160/90, then the doctor considers that the patient has high blood pressure. However, there is a difference in individuals. Without giving consideration to individual condition, statistics may lead to a wrong diagnosis.

The Future of Medicine

Oriental medicine has been giving thought to the mechanism of body movement in relation to the internal organs. Therefore, it tells where to massage in case of heart illness. It tells the stomach is related to a part of the leg, and the eyes are related to another part of the body, etc.

However, even Oriental medicine doesn't tell what kind of movement will give a healing effect on illnesses. This must have been studied by Oriental medicine, but there is no record.

Modern medicine is starting to show an interest in studying Oriental medicine now. It is my opinion that modern medicine must investigate Oriental medicine anatomically, physiologically, histologically, pharmaceutically, chemically, and electromagnetically.

Modern medicine must investigate frankly why Oriental medicine or my sotai exercise cures illness when modern medicine does not. I am not a scholar so I cannot thoroughly explain the mechanism of my exercises. My explanation is simply to make a balance in the body construction. I sincerely wish modern medicine will further investigate the mechanism and the reasons why sotai exercise is effective.

The Principle of Health

Constitution of the Human Body

Basic structure. Man is free to be healthy or sick by his way of living. In other words, he is sick because he does not know what condition maintains health. He is sick because he continues a way of living that eventually brings him illness without his knowing it. However, since we cannot know everything about the cause of sickness, it is important we know the principles of health.

In my opinion, man is a movable building. Let us consider that the four pillars of a four corner house are legs; adding a head and a tail, this will make an animal. When standing up, this animal becomes man (standing on the rear legs of the animal). Because this building moves, construction of the building must be firm and movement must be right. The joints must be movable. It is imaginable from the construction of the body that a movement of one part will cause movement of others. When we neglect this law of movement, we create deformity in our body.

The center of the bones is the spine, which is supported by the pelvis because man stands erect; therefore, the center of our movement is in the waist.

For example, when bending the upper part of the body forward, pull backward at the waist a little, then bend the upper body. This makes bending easier. When bending the upper body to the right, push the waist left and shift the weight on the left leg and then bend. Otherwise bending is difficult. It is not only difficult, but muscle deformity can sometimes be caused.

When exercising the feet, you should stand so that the center of gravity is on your big toe or the inside of the foot.

19

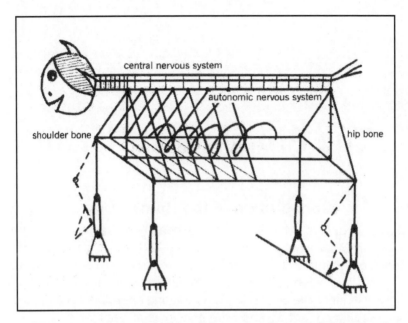

When moving the hand, put force on the small fingers, then press the elbow to the side of the body. This makes force go through the center of the body. In this position, we can have strength. If force is put on the thumb and the elbows are open from the side of the body, we cannot give strength to the arm. Stiffness of the shoulders can result.

The center of our movement is the spine and its base—the pelvis. It is very convenient that the spine is made of short vertebrae. However, because they are put together erect, the spine is easy to deform. Deformities do not often occur in animals whose spines lie horizontal, but it happens more often in man, who stands erect.

When the spine is deformed, irregularity in the autonomic nervous system is caused. Also, muscles attached to the spine create tension, and it causes tension on the nervous system or circulatory system. These are the causes of various sicknesses. Abnormal muscle tension is caused not only by a deformed spine but also by the abuse of certain muscles over a prolonged time.

Four basic activities of life relate to health. Living organisms must adapt to their natural environment; this is absolutely necessary. Due

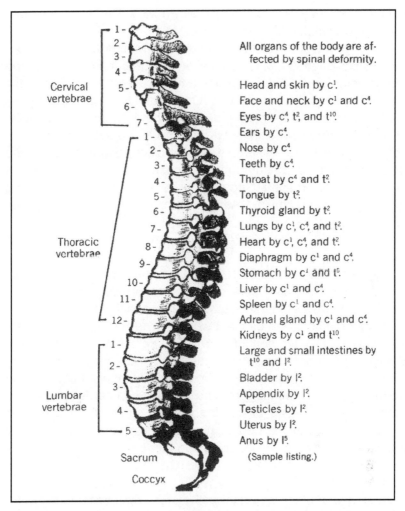

Cervical vertebrae
1-
2-
3-
4-
5-
6-
7-

Thoracic vertebrae
1-
2-
3-
4-
5-
6-
7-
8-
9-
10-
11-
12-

Lumbar vertebrae
1-
2-
3-
4-
5-

Sacrum

Coccyx

All organs of the body are affected by spinal deformity.

Head and skin by c^1.
Face and neck by c^1 and c^4.
Eyes by c^4, t^2, and t^{10}.
Ears by c^4.
Nose by c^4.
Teeth by c^4.
Throat by c^4 and t^2.
Tongue by t^2.
Thyroid gland by t^2.
Lungs by c^1, c^4, and t^2.
Heart by c^1, c^4, and t^2.
Diaphragm by c^1 and c^4.
Stomach by c^1 and t^5.
Liver by c^1 and c^4.
Spleen by c^1 and c^4.
Adrenal gland by c^1 and c^4.
Kidneys by c^1 and t^{10}.
Large and small intestines by t^{10} and l^2.
Bladder by l^2.
Appendix by l^2.
Testicles by l^2.
Uterus by l^2.
Anus by l^5.

(Sample listing.)

to this fact, both nature and living organisms are benefited. However, in reality, living organisms do not adapt to their environment. The reason for this is that living organisms are often out of natural order due to the living style—especially man. He lives according to his knowledge, which often does not conform to natural law.

Man's health is based on breathing, eating and drinking, mental activity, physical movement, and relationship with the environment. In other words, our daily life activities result in our sickness or health. Furthermore, the first four factors are our own activities, and therefore they can be changed as we wish. The condition of our health is the result of our own choice.

If our physical movement causes deformation or stress in our body construction, we will be sick even though our breathing, eating and drinking, and mental activities are right. If we eat wrongly, we will be sick even if we move correctly. These four activities are related to each other. We cannot be healthy by only one right activity.

Under normal conditions, we breathe 17-18 times per minute, women a little more. When we do exercises, breathing becomes faster because we consume more oxygen. On the contrary, when we concentrate on something or worry about something, breathing becomes slow and shallow. As a result, we do deep breathing from time to time.

Living is breathing. Therefore, it is important to know how to breathe for health.

In the Orient, the study of breathing exercise has been highly considered in all fields of artistic study such as judo, fencing, jujitsu, dancing, and tea ceremony—as well as for health improvement.

With breathing, oxygen enters the lungs and permeates the bloodstream. Oxygen combines with red cells in the bloodstream, which in turn supply the whole body's cells with oxygen. The body cell exchanges oxygen and carbon dioxide along with other waste products into the bloodstream. The bloodstream carries carbon dioxide and other waste products screened out by the kidney and throws them out of the body. Thus, breathing is one of the most important activities of living. Breathing can be done unconsciously as well as consciously; therefore, we can improve our breathing by conscious effort.

Eating is another important activity for living. What to eat is indicated by our teeth, their shape and number. We have eight front teeth (4 upper and 4 lower) for cutting vegetables. Four canine teeth are for meat or animal foods. Sixteen back teeth are shaped like grinding stones, good for grains and nuts.

Because teeth are the first place in the body where we acquire our nutrition, I consider that their composition tells us what foods to eat and in what proportion. The composition of teeth indicates that we should eat foods in the above proportions. (See also page 44.)

Any foods, as long as they are natural and whole, can be made

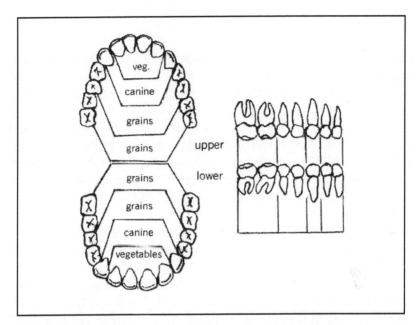

into delicious meals through proper cooking. Chewing is most important. Chewing well, we instinctively want to eat natural and whole foods. Our body in its normal condition is made to accept only natural foods. (For further study of diet, please read macrobiotic books on diet and cooking.)

There is a law for body movement. The first is to move the body in such a way that the center of gravity is always on the waist (the center of the body). In order to do so, put force on the small finger side on the upper body and the big toe side on the lower body. If your shoes wear out on the outside, your walking or action is out of balance. You may become sick; be careful.

To live is a wonderful thing, if we consider even just a few things such as our adaptability to nature's changes, the various functions of metabolism, and the coordination of all the organs. Once you understand the wonderfulness of life, you will reveal gratitude. Life without gratitude is miserable.

Our life is supported by gifts from heaven and earth and the care of parents and others. If we live with thanksgiving for everything provided, our mind is happy and our behavior is kind. As a result, the body becomes sane and healthy. On the other hand, if we are not healthy, our mental activities are not correct.

Design of the human body is perfect. Our body is designed to live happily and healthily. Then why do we become sick? Because we live in a wrong way. We are breaking natural balance by wrong breathing, eating and drinking, body movement, and thinking.

There are several stages of balance in our life. Let the highest balance be 100; health will be over 70; under 70 will be sick. Someone could be 80 on breathing, 60 on diet, 50 on movement, and 90 on thinking. Such a person seems to be happy but will suffer from physical sicknesses. Another could be 70 on breathing, 80 on diet, 80 on movement, but 40 on thinking. He may enjoy physical health and wealth, but he will have many difficulties with his mental activities; he could not be happy. It is desirable to be 100 points in all four activities. However, this is the ideal but not reality.

Some people are more sensitive to their physical balance than others. The body reacts to a physical imbalance immediately and tries to correct it. On the other hand, less sensitive persons react to physical imbalance slowly and sometimes realize the imbalances only after becoming sick. Therefore, one who has sensitivity to physical balance is less prone to sickness. In order to improve the sensitivity, we need conscious activities.

We often make unconscious movements such as yawning, talking to oneself, mental browsing, etc. These movements are examples of the body's unconscious activity towards correcting physical imbalance. Even when we are sleeping, we often move; this movement is also the result of our unconscious activity to correct physical imbalance. There are more imbalances if

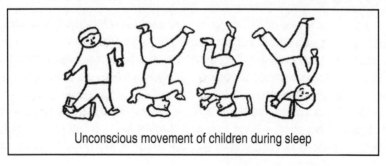

Unconscious movement of children during sleep

one moves a great deal during sleep; a healthy person doesn't move excessively while sleeping. For this reason, it is not advisable to sleep in a soft bed because it makes unconscious movement difficult and physical imbalances will therefore remain uncorrected.

The best application of the unconscious activity is the tickling of children. I used to say that tickling will cure almost all sicknesses of children. Children are so sensitive to tickling that they will try to escape it by any means; this movement corrects any physical imbalance.

For adults, we often cure sicknesses without any medication. We are probably correcting our imbalances unconsciously at these times.

Our senses work delicately. The first judgment as to whether we are sick or healthy will be made by our senses. For example, if the body has something wrong then we have pain, dullness, numbness—generally speaking, abnormal sensations. When we are healthy, we are not aware of any internal organs. However, once we are sick, we become aware of our organs such as the heart, liver, stomach, intestine, eye, ear, etc. We are normally unaware of our eyes; however, once we have trouble with our eyes, we know that our eyes are in front of our face. In other words, we become extremely sensitive when we are sick. This extreme sensitivity is caused by the irregularity of our organs or their functions. However, extreme sensitivity happens well before the beginning of sickness, when there are no symptoms. Therefore, through sensitivity we can know our condition much before modern medicine can diagnose, because modern medicine judges sickness by symptoms.

Because wild animals have good sensitivity (or instinct), they can cure sickness by themselves, or they find and eat grasses that are a natural remedy. However, modern men have lost this instinctive sensitivity: there are more sick people than sick wild animals. Even plants have sensitivity or instinct. For example, corn grows more root when there is a stronger wind. Corn can predict the weather, whether this year has stronger wind or not.

Man does this too. For example, arthritis patients can accurately predict rain because of the increase of pain. If we have good senses that can tell us of very small irregularities in our body, we will be able to correct the imbalance before we become sick. Therefore, it is important to improve our sensitivity.

The Importance of our Movement System

The movement system and sotai. There are two muscle systems in our body. One is smooth muscle and the other is striated muscle. The first one is controlled by the autonomic nervous system; our will cannot activate this system. The latter is the muscle system by which we can move the body by will. Here I am going to discuss this system. (I call it the movement system.)

This movement system (the striated muscle) causes other movements; simultaneously, it holds the body and the internal organs and nerves in place. This movement system consists of bone, cartilage, tendon, muscle, tendon sac, fascia, muscle belt, and skin.

If all the parts move smoothly without any deformations, one is healthy. One muscle relates with other muscles. Therefore, you move one part of the body and the other part also moves more or less. In order to maintain one's health, we must understand the relative movement of all body parts. For this, we have to understand the movement system.

Modern pathology depends on the study of cells or the biochemical character of body fluids, etc. In my opinion, these studies are not enough for maintaining health. The movement system must also be studied. My sotai (healing exercise) is the exercise based on the realization that our body moves as a whole and diseases are the result of accumulated deformations and wrong movements.

The principles of the movement system. For example, lie on your back and move your big toe. If there is no resistance, only the toe moves. However, if you give resistance to the toe movement and try to move the toe, muscles of various parts of the body such as wrists, spine, fingers, neck, face—not only muscles of the same side but also the other side—move too. Because the movement of the toe is connected with other parts of the body such as the hip, spine, and head, we can cure stiff shoulders, headache, tension, deformities, or abnormal arrangement of neck bones, chest bones, and shoulder bones. The 14-meridian system of Chinese medicine is the result of the acknowledgment of the interrelationship of these muscles.

Sometimes abnormal places are hidden so that we only realize them by pressing with our fingers or by moving the joints; for example, sometimes we feel better after giving massage on a particular part of the body. This means there is stress on this spot and by removing this stress the muscle returns to normal. Ticklish feeling and pain by touching mean that some different grades of stress exist.

Good posture is advisable. However, if we correct someone's posture forcefully we may cause physical imbalance. When we have bad posture, such as one side of the shoulder is up or the neck is tilted to one side, we are balanced in this posture. In other words, our spine is straighter, breathing is smoother, action is smoother. Correcting the posture may cause pain and difficulty in body movement, including movements of internal organs. Therefore, in order to correct the posture, we must correct the cause of the bad posture.

If there is deformity in a joint, there is an imbalance in that joint and, therefore, stress in the muscles that are connected to that joint. Stretch, turn, pull, and push that joint from one side to the other. You will find that one side is easier than the other. Then another person should move the joint in the easier direction, and at the same time you give resistance to that movement. When the resistance reaches high, let him relax suddenly. This will take off stress and help to correct a deformation of bones or joints.

For example, you may experience that your neck cannot turn in the morning due to a bad position while sleeping. At such a time, try to move the neck forward, backward, left, right, up, down; find out which is easiest, then ask someone to give resistance to your movement as you move your neck in the easiest direction. When resistance reaches the limit, then relax suddenly. Many abnormal joints or muscle deformities can be cured by this.

If you are alone, you can apply the same principle to correcting joints. If you have pain at the waist, stand up with natural form and turn or bend forward, backward, left, right, up and down. Find out the easiest movement. Practice the easiest motion several times.

Most training asks us to force difficult movements. Actually, this kind of training has no benefit to our health—it might even be harmful. Comfortable movement is the right movement; it is natural law. Rehabilitative therapy should know this law.

When you do the correcting motion, the important thing is the selection of the joint to be used for the resistance motion.

Within the many joints—hand, elbow, foot, knee, neck, spine, bottom of the spine, shoulder—the joint of the legs and the lower body is most important. The body weight is supported by the buttocks. If the body is not balanced at this joint, you will create stress all over the body. Therefore, any good movement you may do at the periphery of the body is no use if the balance at the waist is not corrected.

Another important thing is that the center of gravity should be on the center line of the body. For this, Japanese fencing (kendo) teaches to hold the sword with the small finger tight so that both arms turn inward. By such holding, movement of the arms should be gathered at the center line of the body; this posture will create the strongest power. If you try to use the sword with open arms, you cannot cut anything because your body strength is not centralized.

In golfing as well as fencing, your knees should be inward so that the center of gravity lies on the center line. To do this, Japanese martial arts teach us that we should stand using the big toes. This makes our center of gravity follow the body's center line. All exercises should be done in this manner, otherwise we will be tired easily and have bodily imbalance. Breathing from the hara (abdomen) or holding one's breath in the hara has the same effect, and this is emphasized in Japanese martial arts.

All exercises that are not done under the condition that the center of gravity is on the center line of the body cause imbalance in the movement system. On the other hand, if the center of gravity is on the center line, it cures imbalance existing in the movement system. Otherwise, one becomes tired easily. Also, all turning motion should use the waist as a pivot. One who does exercises, yoga, or tai-chi must know this fact. By the same reason, weightlifting may straighten the imbalance.

Usually one leg is longer than the other. One can compare this by putting the two ankles together. This results from the fact that we usually put the center of gravity to one side more often than the other side.

For example, many people are right handed; therefore, they pick something up from the floor with the right hand. At this time, many people put the right foot forward and bend. In this case, the center of gravity is on the right side of the body and not on the center. If you constantly repeat such motion, your right side will grow more than the left side. This motion is very awkward compared with keeping the left foot forward; the latter places the center of gravity at the center of the body and makes the motion smooth and stable. This is the way of natural movement. When we violate this natural movement we will cause deformation in some part of the body, especially in the spine.

Most right handed persons have their pelvis tilted toward the right front and the left leg joint slides backward. This causes the left side of the body to tighten and the right side to lengthen. Therefore, the left knee becomes tight, the left chest thickens, and the left shoulder becomes tight. Such imbalance will cause further troubles. The right handed person should step forward with the left foot and then bend. In this way, he can balance left and right and can avoid accidental falling or twisting. Watch a baseball pitcher. He steps forward with the left leg and then the right hand goes forward, leaving the left foot behind. His center of gravity moves on the same line from backward to forward.

In the same way, our muscles are tight on one side and loose on the other side. If one side is always tight and never loosened, it will suffer. Our muscles must be alternately tight and loose.

We breathe unconsciously. However, we have to exhale or inhale consciously when we do fast or special actions. Never make quick movements when inhaling. In martial arts, the fighter finds the time to attack when the opponent inhales. In martial arts or athletics, one should inhale quickly and exhale slowly. Therefore, in the sotai exercises; we recommend quick inhale and slow exhale. This is the secret of all chanting, meditation, and breathing methods of ancient or present health practices.

Turn Sick Body to Healthy Body

What is sickness? What is health? Living things adapt to their natural environment. This is the absolute order; however, in reality this often does not happen so people become sick. The reason for this is that the daily way of life is out of order. People have been taught many healthy ways of living in the past; all of them have some benefit but lack in the overall validity.

Principles of Diagnosis and Restoring Health

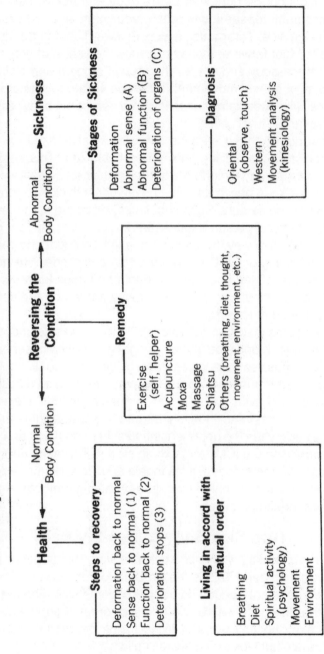

Health — Normal Body Condition → Reversing the Condition → Abnormal Body Condition → Sickness

Steps to recovery

Deformation back to normal
Sense back to normal (1)
Function back to normal (2)
Deterioration stops (3)

Living in accord with natural order

Breathing
Diet
Spiritual activity (psychology)
Movement
Environment

Remedy

Exercise (self, helper)
Acupuncture
Moxa
Massage
Shiatsu
Others (breathing, diet, thought, movement, environment, etc.)

Stages of Sickness

Deformation
Abnormal sense (A)
Abnormal function (B)
Deterioration of organs (C)

Diagnosis

Oriental (observe, touch)
Western
Movement analysis (kinesiology)

adapting to the environment

losing adaptation to the environment

There are four factors of absolute necessity for living: breathing; eating and drinking (diet); body movement; and mental activity. Everyone must have these four factors for living. These factors are related to each other. The environment influences them all.

When these factors become out of order, it causes stress on the muscles. This causes further sensory abnormality, and sickness then follows. Acupuncture cures many sicknesses by stimulating the pressure points. These cures are caused by relaxing tension by stimulating the points. In my opinion, the tension of tissue creates internal pressure, which causes pain by stimulating the nerves. Acupuncture relieves tension and cures sickness. In other words, tension causes sickness.

What is the cause of excess stress on the tissues or muscles?

The main cause is stress in the muscles that connect to the bones over the joints. If excessive stress is put on the muscle, this will make bone deformities: if the bones are put under excessive stress, this will make muscle deformities.

In other words, deformed joints cause the deformation of muscles that are connected to the bones. This deformation disturbs the nervous system and the circulatory system. This will cause sensory abnormalities such as pain, feeling poor, tiredness. This is a warning sign of sickness—the first warning of sickness (A). If deformation continues, malfunctioning of the organs will begin (B). The further this develops, the more deterioration of the organs will start (C).

At this stage, the doctor can give the name of the disease or a diagnosis of the disease. The process of sickness is A to B (includes A) to C (includes A and B). This process is reversible. If deformation diminishes, the body will go back to its normal condition. In this case, abnormality of the senses will return to normal (1). Recovery of the malfunction of the organs follows (2). Finally, the deterioration of the organs will be cured (3).

However, the cure for this deterioration is limited. If the deterioration has gone too far, there is no cure for it.

A wrong way of thinking—"to cure such and such diseases." It is wrong to say, "I am ill because my organs are unhealthy." You should say, "My organs are unhealthy because my body is unhealthy." In other words, the basic body structure is deformed, causing pain in the hips or poor feeling. This is stage A.

If this continues, the organs will worsen and become bad. For example, diarrhea or constipation (malfunction of the stomach) may result. This stage is B. If this malfunctioning continues further, then we have deterioration of the stomach such as an ulcer, stage C. People think an ulcer causes severe pain. In reality, this is backward. First, we have deformation in the body; then, if this deformation progresses, it will result in the ulcer. In other words, sickness comes first, then damage to the organs. Damaged organs are not causing the sickness. *The damaged organs are the result of body deformation.*

For example, in curing an ulcerated stomach, start by correcting deformations. The first result is feeling better. Then the stomach function will become better. Then the ulcer will heal. This is the process of healing stomach ulcers.

Most persons do not think this way. If a person has an ulcer in his stomach, he probably would try to cure the ulcer first. If you are not feeling good, you go to a medical doctor who will look for a bad organ; he may find an ulcerated stomach. Then he would try to fix this ulcer. If there is no ulcer in the stomach and the function of the stomach is not bad, the doctor cannot help you. In such cases, the doctor will tell you that you are overworked, you need rest, or you are nervous.

Correcting deformation is healing. Future medicine must study deformation of the body and correction of the deformation.

Secrets of correcting deformation. Because our bodies were originally healthy, we feel good when we are returning to this original condition. Therefore, avoid painful movements. If our movement is easy or smooth, we are going back to our originally healthy condition. Man is made in such a way that he can move his joints easily and avoid hard movement. Unconsciously, we are making easy movements. By this easy movement, we are instinctively correcting deformation. This is the principle of my sotai exercise. If you understand this principle, you can cure your illness.

If you have pain when you move your hand to the left, try to move it to the right. If this is easier than the left, then the right side movement is curing the deformation. Up and down, front and back—

do the same thing.

The human body was originally made healthy, then deformation made sickness. Correcting this deformation is curing. To correct deformation, all you need is easy movement instead of painful, forced movement. This is the secret of sotai exercise and the secret of health. However, if your life is disorderly, this deformation will start again.

There are several ways to correct deformations. Drugs, acupuncture, or moxibustion may be effective. Some people may be corrected one way or another; you may need another way. It is a personal choice as to which method to use in curing oneself. Any technique is useful if it brings one to the original, healthy condition. Therefore, don't stick stubbornly to one method or a rigid technique.

Correcting deformation by oneself is better than being corrected by others. When the spine is deformed, the muscles around the spine become tense and put pressure or tension on nerves or blood vessels. As a result, we have pains in the back, waist, ribs, chest, abdomen, etc. There are many techniques for correcting spinal deformations. One of them is the chiropractic method. However, this requires a high skill. If a chiropractor is not very skillful, treatment may worsen the condition. There are many such cases even with skilled practitioners. However, in this sotai exercise you decide movement toward the direction that makes you feel better, and you never force painful movement. Therefore, sotai exercise never worsens the condition.

Shiatsu is another technique for curing deformation. This is curing tense muscles caused by deformed bone connections by applying finger, palm, or foot pressure. When muscle tension is eliminated, bone connections return to normal and sickness will be cured.

This technique also requires high skill, and it is not always easy to find such persons. If the pressures are applied wrongly, deformations may increase. With sotai exercise, you do this yourself. You always know if you applied the wrong force. Therefore, you cannot make a mistake with sotai exercise.

Health should be maintained by oneself. Doctors just give guidance. Only you can maintain your health. Many doctors have misunderstood in believing that they cured such and such disease. They merely took away the pain. However, pain is an important warning sign that helps us to avoid a more serious illness. Therefore, taking away pain without curing the cause of the pain may lead to a serious illness. When you have pain, you must correct the cause of the pain instead of just removing it. Doctors remove the pain, but it is you who corrects the cause of the pain.

Most patients rely on doctors, believing the doctor cures sickness. They are dependent. Such persons have difficulty being healthy. They may be cured temporarily; however, they will be sick again soon. Buddha said that ignorance is the worst disease. In my opinion, sickness is the result of living against natural law. This is ignorance of natural law.

Health Maintenance

Self Health Check-up

In most cases, pains in legs, waist, back, etc. are caused by deformation of nerves or blood vessels. These deformations are caused by muscle tensions or pressures which are caused by spinal deformations. The deformation of nerves or blood vessels eventually causes illness in the internal organs. Therefore, the first stage of sickness is the deformation of the spine as well as the whole body movement system.

Therefore, all deformations of the movement system should be corrected soon. However, we often are not aware of this deformation. The deformations can be seen from the outside, but it is difficult to see this by ourselves. We are only aware of it when deformation causes pain. However, there is a way to detect this by ourselves. Because deformation appears not only in shape but also in movement, we can detect deformations by movement.

The easiest way to find deformation is to move the muscle joints such as the joints of the legs, knees, hands, elbows, shoulders, and hips. There are only four movements of these joints:

a) Moving the joints back and forth.
b) Moving the joints left and right.
c) Twisting the joints left and right.
d) Contracting and loosening the joints.

We check the joints to see which are difficult to move and which direction is more difficult to move. Then exercise only the joints which are not difficult to move and only in the direction that is *not difficult*. Three to five times for each movement will be enough to loosen up hard joints.

Method of self check-up.

(a) A 'top' movement

Knees on the floor.
Toes touching the floor.
Heels supporting the buttocks.
Hands on the heels.

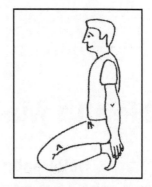

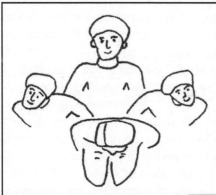

Relax the shoulders, pivoting the upper part of the body on the hips, keeping the hands on the heels, 3 times clockwise and 3 times counterclockwise. (While pivoting move as far right, forward, left, and backward as possible—like a spinning top.)

Almost all the joints will move by this exercise, so that by this movement we can check which joints are deformed or stiff. After finding the more difficult direction, give movement to the easier side 3 to 5 times.

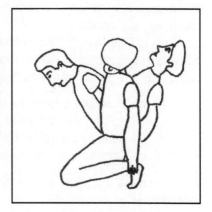

(b) Crawling movement

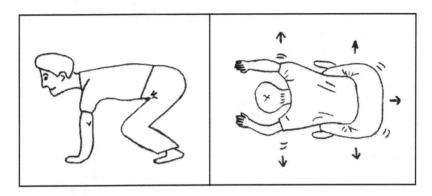

Both hands and feet on the floor, knees not touching the floor. Move the buttocks and shoulders from left to right and back and forth. If you find it difficult to move one direction or some joint, then that direction or joint has deformation. So give movement to the easier side 3 to 5 times.

(c) Swinging buttocks movement

Stand against a wall, put hands on the wall at eye level and support the body. Bend knees, not touching each other. Swing hips from left to right, then from right to left, finding the more difficult side. Move 2 or 3 times more toward the easier side. Make sure all parts of the body are relaxed when movements are made.

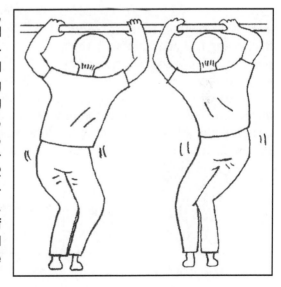

Good or Bad Posture

Posture can tell us if we are in good health or if we are sick.

Before we can do this, we have to improve our observation so that we can judge posture that is good and that which is not. The position of the shoulders and neck makes one's posture look good or bad. Fashions are changing; some styles are healthy, some are not. A healthy style encourages a straight backbone. Stand with the back against the wall—head, shoulders, and hips touching the wall. Put either your right or left hand behind you between your back and the wall, leaving space (enough for your hand). Heels of the feet about 1 inch from the wall. Back of the knees not touching the wall. If you can stand in this position comfortably, you are in pretty good shape. If you are not comfortable in this position, there is some deformation in the area that is uncomfortable.

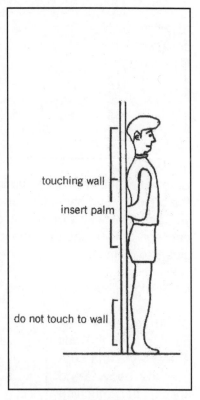

In order to create good posture, you have to correct your feet first. Stand with the soles of the feet evenly touching the floor, putting your weight on the center of the feet (*sokushin*).

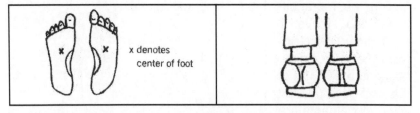

Most people stand on the outside part of the heel. These people walk slow and their actions are slow. Shoes wear down on the outside part of the heel. People who wear out the front soles of their shoes are short tempered; they are quick and more active. The ideal type is wearing down the soles evenly.

To make standing even, do the following exercise: Standing, feet parallel, hands on the kneecaps, knees bent slightly, swing the hips from left to right and from right to left. If you find that one side is more difficult to move than the other, swing hips to the easier side 4 or 5 more times.

Men and women have different bone structure. Women have bigger hips because the pelvic structure is larger. This is an advantage for women to conceive and for the growth of the baby. Men's shoulders are wider, so men are more fit to do work with their arms. Men often have stiff shoulders from heavy work. The cause of stiffness in the shoulders is the misuse of force. Place the elbows close to the body and let the force pass through the small finger side. Then you will get the most power from your hand without stiffening your shoulders.

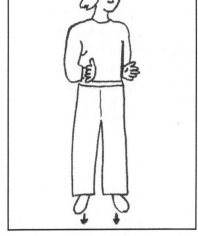

Sitting in *seiza* (Japanese style of sitting with knees bent and feet tucked under) position is best. If you can sit in this position for a long time, you are in pretty good shape. If you can sit in this position with your backbone straight, then you will live a long life. If you are sitting in this position and your back is not straight, then you have reached old age even though you are still young. If the chin is forward, you are tired.

Body posture changes with your emotions; emotions are related to posture.

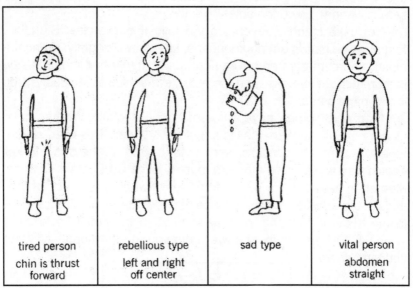

tired person	rebellious type	sad type	vital person
chin is thrust forward	left and right off center		abdomen straight

Body and mind are front and back. The center of the body is the waist. Therefore, if we move the body with the center of gravity at the waist, our movement is most smooth, beautiful, and graceful. All Japanese martial arts, dancing, and other trainings teach this.

Look at someone's posture when he is crying: the head is down, the abdomen is weak, the backbone is bent like an old man. If you have this posture, you will get a sad feeling. The body and mind are related to each other.

Another example: 'to be angry at' in Japanese means straightening of the abdomen. In other words, when you are angry, your abdomen is straightened and tense. This overstimulates the liver functions and sometimes damages the liver. Therefore, Chinese medicine relates anger to the liver.

Emotions change breathing. When you are nervous, you breathe with the chest and the chest becomes tense. When you relax, the abdomen is strengthened. Therefore, a person who can laugh even when he is troubled is a person who can relax his chest and have strength in his abdomen. If you laugh by loud voicing, the abdomen is stressed and the parasympathetic nerve will be stimulated. You will be able to calm down. You will be able to balance your emotions.

Three Secrets of Right Movement

Balanced, smooth movement is beautiful. Dancing is an art. It is beautiful when its movement is balanced. When movement is balanced, the center of gravity is resting on *kikai*, three fingers below the navel. If the center of gravity is higher than kikai, the movement is not balanced; it is no longer beautiful and it is easy to become tired. (Kikai is positioned at about the 3rd lumbar vertebra.)

Rules of smooth movements. The other day, a ping-pong player came to my clinic because he was not feeling good. He played ping-pong using his right hand with his weight on his right foot. He thought this was the right position, but the movement was not smooth. Because of his bad form, he was creating discomfort.

Let us see how four-legged animals crawl. When their right front leg moves forward, the left rear leg moves forward at the same time. When the left front leg moves forward, the right rear leg moves forward at the same time. Moving legs like this, the center of gravity stays at the center of their body.

Men stand erect and walk. However, the movement of the arms and legs should be the same. When the left leg (rear leg) moves forward, the right arm (front leg) moves forward. When the right leg (rear leg) moves forward, the left arm (front leg) moves forward. Walking like this we are keeping the center of gravity at the center of the body all the time.

Similarly, when you use the right hand, you should put your weight on the left foot.

If you are right-handed, you use your right hand to pick up things. So try to see which side, left or right, is easier for the feet to support weight. Also, find out on which foot you put more weight when cutting vegetables. One day I asked the chef of a famous restaurant, "What kind of posture do you take when cutting vegetables?" He said, "I pull back on the right foot, so my weight is on the left foot. In this position, I can cut accurately." Not only chefs, anyone working with his hands should keep a balance of his hands and feet.

If using the right hand, the body weight must be on the left foot. If we do not balance left and right, this will cause us to be tired, with pain in the back and waist. The center of gravity must move with our movement.

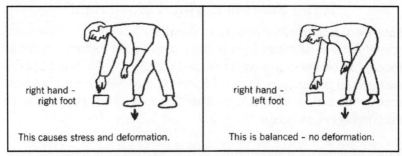

In conclusion: When bending to the left (right), the weight moves towards the right (left). When bending forward (backward), weight should be moved to the buttock (forward). When stretching your hand to reach up high, you move your weight up. When twisting your body, your body weight moves towards the twisting direction.

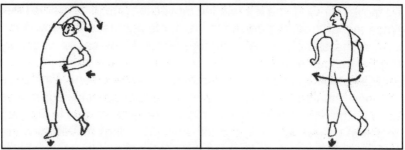

How to do exercises. For health, people try many sports or exercises. However, most people do not realize that wrong movement of the body causes unhealthy conditions or damage to the muscles. One must realize that good exercise is different from hard training. Many sportsmen practice hard training in order to win the game. This is not good exercise and is sometimes dangerous.

Body muscles are constructed in pairs such as left and right, front and back, and up and down. If one side is deformed, hard training increases this deformity. Therefore, the good exercise first corrects deformity and then develops muscles evenly on both sides.

In other words, if muscle movement has resistance, that muscle has deformations. Then, we have to move in the other direction, which has no resistance. When this direction is exercised, the muscle will be relaxed, and you can exercise the other direction without resistance. This is the good exercise that will improve muscle strength. Exercise without this adjustment can damage or injure muscles.

At present, jogging, dancing, exercising, and all kinds of sports are popular. This is a result of overnourishment or overeating. It is a way to burn up the extra calorie intake. However, if exercises are done without balancing or smoothing out deformities, they will be injurious to the body.

Breathing Exercise

Breathing for longevity. A good breathing exercise gives us longevity. The easiest kind of breathing exercise is done in bed before sleep.

Use no pillow. Put both hands on the lower abdomen, legs straight, knees touching, feet a little apart, toes facing inward a little. Then start to exhale. This must be done by movement of the diaphragm. Contract the abdomen—then air goes out from the lungs. Completely and slowly, the air comes from the lungs. Then you inhale very automatically. This is very natural movement. Therefore, exhaling is the important thing—the inhale follows naturally. Exhaling moves the backbone in a curved position and inhaling moves it straight. Therefore, deep breathing makes a backbone exercise.

Continue the breathing exercise and try for a period to exhale longer. Around the 10th day, you may breathe less than 2 to 3 times per minute. Less breathing means bigger lung capacity and long life. Please try this exercise every night. If you do better breathing, you are improving your health every moment because you have to breathe every moment all your life.

Deep breathing for psychology. Nightly exercise of breathing will improve abdominal power. When we have strength in the abdomen, we can move fast, don't become upset, get work done, and have decision power to overcome difficulties.

When breathing is around the chest, the orthosympathetic nervous system is stimulated and one becomes nervous. Contrarily, if strength is in the abdomen, the parasympathetic nerve is stimulated, and we are less nervous and have control power. Therefore, when we do deep breathing exercise, we improve our psychological mode.

Thanks to breathing. One of the most important exercises is pushing around the abdomen just before sleep. At the same time, give appreciation to the existence of breathing, without which we cannot live a moment. Then we can sleep very deeply, because appreciation will bring relaxation to our mentality and nervous system.

Foods for Health

Simple and light. Dr. S. Kondo, Honorary Professor of Tohoku University, researched all over Japan to find the causes of longevity and short life. The following is one of his reports.

He found a village where there were many short lives due to heart disease. Curiously enough, he noticed that the next villagers were lacking heart disease. Further research revealed an interesting fact. The next villagers were descendants of the Heike clan, which was defeated by the Genji clan several hundred years ago. Because they were not allowed to catch fish, they lived by vegetarianism. Grains, vegetables, beans, and seaweeds were their foods. From this example, we learn that we will have a better heart condition eating without fish and other animal foods.

According to statistics for the first, second, and third generations of Japanese in Hawaii, South America, and North America, heart disease and arterial disease are increasing as animal food consumption increases.

Many of my patients think that animal foods have a better nutritional value than other nutrients. Therefore, they believe they should eat animal foods as much as possible. As a result, they are trying to eat fish, eggs, and even beef every day. This is a grand mistake. Those people's bodies are so stiff that they can't bend easily. If they don't change their diet, there is no medicine that will cure them.

In our jaw, man has 4 canine teeth, which is 1/7 the number of our total teeth; these are for meat. We have 8 teeth designed for cutting vegetables, which is 2/7 of the total. Finally, we have 16 teeth for grinding grains, which is 4/7 of the total teeth. Therefore, according to our tooth structure, our proportion of food should be 4/7 grains, 2/7 vegetables, and 1/7 animal foods.

Wild animals consume foods they catch in the field. They naturally eat seasonal and local food. When agriculture and transportation were not as developed as today, man was also consuming foods that were available from his environment. Due to the development of transportation and refrigeration techniques, we can eat foods in off seasons, such as vegetables made in vinyl houses (hothouses), and foods imported from far away, which are often loaded with preservatives. We should ask ourselves, isn't this expansion of food habits the cause of much increase in degenerative diseases such as heart disease, arteriosclerosis, and cancer?

Another important point we should consider is that whole foods are much more nutritious than partial or refined foods. The modern food market supplies many food supplements, because they sell mostly partial or refined foods, which lack many important nutrients. It is doubtful, however, that merely adding food supplements will bring back the food's value to equal the original value.

Whole foods have life force and partial foods have none. Adding supplements to partial or refined foods does not give foods the life force that only nature, not man, can create. Therefore, small whole fish is better than pieces of big fish. Brown rice is better than white rice, which lacks the budding part of the rice. In other words, brown rice will grow if given water and sunshine, but white rice will not. Why did we get the idea that the whiter the rice, the better it is? (This is a popular idea in Japan.)

Agriculture makes the foundation of health. Food is the source of life. Therefore, it is obvious that the kind of food we produce is the most important factor for our health. If we grow weak grains or vegetables, don't we become weak physically? Then, we have to consider what kind of agriculture makes grains or vegetables weak. Wild grasses or mountain vegetables are so strong that they survive in snow or bad weather. But if we transplant them in our gardens and add fertilizers and insecticides, they become weak and die. Does this mean that agriculture is making weaker or inferior produce?

When Dr. Takakura returned from the war front, he was worried about the use of DDT because he did research on poisonous gas in the Japanese army. He studied the effects of DDT and other insecticides. Then when all the farmers were happy with the use of insecticides because they had the best crops in their life, Dr. Takakura warned about their use. Now people are realizing his foresight.

There are many problems to study in agriculture, not only insecticides. Future agriculture has to develop so that the farmer can make produce for better health, not better money.

Warning for mothers. Dr. Kondo, a researcher of longevity, once said that there is no special evidence that fruits are especially good for health. Furthermore, we must realize the fact that many farmers and neighbors are suffering from the use of insecticides for growing apples. Foods recommended by nutritional science have been reconsidered now.

Consumers, especially mothers, must select their foods so that families can maintain health. Mothers should find the best foods for their families.

My fasting. I often heard that fasting has a good effect on health. In order to confirm this idea, I fasted for 10 days with eleven people; 4 girl students of mine, 1 boy (about 20 years old), 2 government workers, 2 people around 50 years old, and 1 of 65 years. I was 70.

The first 2 days, we ate half of our regular amount of food. Then we fasted for 10 days. We took 6 days to return to normal eating.

During the fasting time, we drank I cup of honey water (1 teaspoonful honey in 1 cup water) and 1 cup of vegetable juice. When we felt weak, we drank ume-sho-ban (1 umeboshi, 1/4 teaspoon ginger, 1 teaspoon soy sauce, and hot bancha tea).

During this time we got up at 5 o'clock and did deep breathing, *zazen* meditation, exercise, and running (about 1.5 miles). Then we took cold showers and went to our own jobs. After returning home from work we did exercise, breathing, and *zazen* meditation. Like this, we worked 3 times more than normal and were never tired. By this fasting, all of us learned that 10 days fasting will not reduce our energy but rather increase it. This was a surprising experience for us all.

Practical Suggestions for Sotai Treatment

General Suggestions

How to move. In order to apply sotai treatments, a helper must lead the patient so that he moves all his body parts. If there is a malady in some part, that part is especially difficult to move. A skillful helper can move such parts. This is the key point in determining who is a good helper.

After all parts move, we find the direction that is easiest to move. Then let the patient move the parts in the easier direction. It is important to decide how far he has to move parts of the body. At a certain point, the treatment giver should stop that movement, and give resistance. After resistance, build up and release quickly. To find this point is the most important factor. Too much movement or not enough movement—in either case the treatment will not bring the best results. You will know this point after much experience. In the beginning, however, you had better ask the patient. If he feels pain, he has moved too much—so he has to stop movement before such a point.

The next important thing is how to move the waist. All our movements relate to the waist. Therefore, when he relaxes his feet, he has to relax the waist. And if he moves the feet, he has to move from the waist.

Another thing you have to remember is that you have to position the patient so that he can relax his whole body. If some parts of the body have stress, sotai treatment doesn't work. For this, the best position is lying down. When the patient is lying down, his arms should stretch alongside his body. If they stretch out above the head, or are placed under the chin, it causes stress and strain. You have to watch such details in order to get good results.

The most important sotai treatments. Sotai treatment starts from the legs. Deformation of the legs is the beginning of deformation. Treatment of the legs alone can correct half the deformation of the body.

For the legs, the first treatment is the knees—see sotai exercise 15, page 78.

In exercise 15, if the left leg has pain, give treatment on the left leg. If both legs have pain, give treatment on both sides. The angle of the knee is about 90 degrees. The patient (**A**) should bend his toes by raising his foot. This has an effect on the whole muscle. If this treatment does not reduce pain in the knee, try again after bending the knee sharper. The next treatment is also on the leg (see exercises 21 and 22). If a patient has too much pain to bend his leg, give treatment to the other leg that has less pain. (Exercise 21 gives treatment on the leg that is more difficult to bend.) If one has no pain when he is bending his legs, give exercise 23, followed by exercises 24, 25, & 26.

Also you can give the following treatment, which was not mentioned in the exercise section of this book: **B** (helper) bends or twists the upper body of **A** (patient) to the left and right from the back while **A** is sitting on a chair. If there is any uncomfortable movement, let **A** move his upper body from harder side to easier side like all other remedy exercises.

Relieving Pains

Migraine headache. In this case, one usually has a deformation in the neck (cervical spine). You can find a painful point on the neck using your finger. While touching with finger, try to move your neck, shoulder, upper body, and waist so that the pains go away. If one cannot find the painful spot by oneself, ask another to apply pressure to the neck area. At this time, one should lie on one's back on the floor so that relaxation is easier. Also try exercise 28, page 96.

Stiff neck in the morning. The cause of this trouble is prolonged bad posture of the neck. It usually results from watching TV or reading a book, magazine, or newspaper with bad posture.

First bend the neck front and back, turn left and right, and bend to left and right. Find out which one is most painful. After finding the most painful point, **A** moves neck toward opposite direction (no pain direction). **B** (helper) gives resistance as **A** moves neck while exhaling. Then stop (inhale). Hold the breath a few seconds and exhale quickly. This time **A** should relax completely. If once is not enough try 2-3 times.

Pains in neck, shoulders, and arm. Try exercises 24, 26, 33, 34, 35.

Old age shoulder pain. Mostly this pain comes from the feet. Try exercises 15 and 27. Also try exercises 24 and 33. This is difficult to treat. Experience is required.

Hip pains. We often experience pain in the hips. Medical doctors take X-rays. If the hip bone or vertebrae are not injured, they will say to just rest. Even if they find problems with the vertebrae, they say there is no way to cure.

These pains are caused by muscle tissue putting too much pressure on the nerves. Curing those pains requires finding movement that alleviates the pain and repeating such exercises.

A good exercise for hip pains is basic exercise 3. Bend the upper body forward and backward. Find out which direction has no pain. Then repeat, bending toward only this direction. Five or six times of this exercise will much reduce the pain. Test bending the other way. If there is still pain, exercise another 5-6 times in the same way at another time. Also try exercises 16, 22, 30.

One time two soccer players came to my clinic. They claimed pain in the hips. I asked them to lie on their stomach and bend the legs. They could not touch the buttocks with their feet. They felt pain if I pushed the feet closer to the buttocks. In the same position I applied exercise 23 (or 45) and their troubles were cured immediately.

Foot pains. When the feet have problems, the whole body has problems. Our feet support the entire body. Therefore, it is important that the feet touch the ground evenly. Check the soles of your shoes. If they are worn flat, your condition is good. However, most people wear out the heel or the outside of the heel first. When shoes are not wearing evenly, the knee will be deformed. Deformed knees will cause deformation of the thigh joints which will in turn deform the hip bone. Finally, the spine will be deformed.

Therefore, it is a very serious condition if one has pain in the feet and knees. When there is pain in the feet or knees, move the joints of the feet and knees in all directions, and find the direction which has no pain. That is the direction you have to apply sotai exercises.

Sicknesses of Internal Organs

Stomachache. When children claim stomachache, mothers often don't know what to do. Don't panic. Apply palm over the abdomen (see exercise 39). The palm radiates infrared rays that can often cure stomachaches. In case of infants, give ticklings on the side of the abdomen. If there is much pain, apply exercise 40. Also exercise 16 will be good. When applying exercise 40, one can push hard even though the patient claims it is very painful.

Gastroptosis. The best exercise for this is to lie on the back, stretch out both legs and try to lift the heels up from the floor. Keep that position for a few seconds at first. As you exercise more, prolong the time to 1-2 minutes, raising the heels higher at the same time. If one side is more difficult than the other, try the easier side. Exercises 17 and 42 will also be good.

Palpitation of the heart. Because the nerves controlling the heart (para- and orthosympathetic nerves) are passing through the muscles of the neck or ribs, if those muscles are deformed it will cause an abnormal condition in the heart function. This is one of the causes of heart palpitation.

Modern Western medicine overlooks this muscular deformation. Therefore, unfortunately, their treatments are often ineffective. Contrary to Western medicine, Oriental medicine has been developed in this area and has been giving treatments for deformations with good results for a long time. This is one of the reasons Oriental medicine remained in Japan when Western medicine was authorized by her government.

The deformation of muscle cannot be detected by electrocardiogram, and people often have to worry as to what is the cause of their palpitation. This palpitation is often caused by gas pressure that has fermented inside the large intestine. If this gas happens on the left side, it pushes the heart; if on the right side, it pushes the liver. As a result, many physical malfunctions or bad feelings happen. In such cases, sickness is gas formation in the large intestine and not really in the heart or liver.

Asthma. A concave sternum often causes this. The junctions of the ribs and vertebrae may have deformities. Apply basic sotai exercises with helper (14-26, pages 75-94).

Blood pressure. The reason for high blood pressure is the heart is working with extra effort in order to circulate blood. The cause of this is very simple. The flow of blood is disturbed. How? The blood is too sticky and/or the blood vessels become too narrow; this is caused by deposits of the famous cholesterol. If one changes the blood condition (less sticky), the pressure will be lowered.

Low blood pressure means the heart is weak. Taking drugs without correcting the cause is meaningless. In my opinion, measuring the grade of health by blood pressure is a mistake, because someone may be very healthy having adapted to a higher than normal blood pressure.

If one observes the basic sotai exercises, both self and helper, the blood pressure will become normal as one's body becomes more balanced.

Persons with a red face, oily face, high blood pressure, and short temper have bad blood circulation. Those people may have strokes. The opposite of this is the case of frigidity. This is also caused by bad circulation. Check for abnormalities of the spine and hip bone.

(Translator's note: From the macrobiotic view concerning the above heart troubles, the macrobiotic diet should be observed. For this, please read macrobiotic books written by George Ohsawa, Michio Kushi, Herman Aihara, Cornellia Aihara, etc.)

Other Sicknesses

Dizziness. This can be caused by subluxation of the 3rd thoracic vertebra. Apply exercise 29.

Insomnia. This is often caused by hardening of the upper neck muscles. Finger massage on this part is good, as well as applications of sotai exercise. Give exercise 31.

Neuralgia. In most cases of neuralgia, there is nothing wrong with the nerves. The pain comes from our sensorial nerve. Something stimulates the sensorial nerve, and we feel pain. The causes of the stimulation are sometimes chemical, physical, or psychological. Sometimes it is environmental, such as pressure or wind. In any case, in my opinion, the cause of stimulation is bodily deformation. Determine painful movement and apply opposite movement.

Facial neuralgia. Deformations may exist in the brain or skull. However, the cause of the deformation of the skull may be in other places. Check all body movement, starting from the feet. If you find an easy movement, then apply sotai exercises as mentioned previously.

Common cold. Apply exercise 38 or 15.

Women's Diseases

Disease of women's sexual organs. Because the female sexual organ is located in the pelvis, the cause of women's disease is often the deformation of the pelvis. Medical doctors usually look at the sexual organs but not at the pelvis, which is causing the sickness. Therefore, after operations, the same sickness often happens again. Correcting the deformation of the pelvis not only cures women's diseases but also cures the inability to conceive.

People say whether one has an easier delivery or not depends on how big the pelvis is. However, in my opinion, the improper connection between the pelvis and the sacrum is the real cause.

Let the patient lie on the back and then the abdomen, and move her legs skillfully. Often the deformations are corrected. By this, I cured many menstrual troubles, possible loss of a baby, and women's sicknesses. I even cured a lady who had an upside-down fetus.

Breast hardness. One way to check for breast cancer is to test whether there is a hard muscle in the breast or not. However, existence of hard muscle in the breast is not always a sign of cancer. Giving good sotai exercise (29, 34, and 35) often loosens up those hard muscles.

Infant and Baby Care

Parents are responsible for infants' sickness. There are children often coming to me due to difficult hearing. The cause of this is often due to medications taken by the mother during her pregnancy. There are also nearsightedness, abnormal bending of spine, allergy, and cancer. Mother's breathing, diet, movements, and emotional thinking are responsible for these.

To move the body to the easier side is the secret of the sotai remedy. However, infants can't tell us which side is easier or difficult. Therefore, the best way to apply sotai exercise to an infant is to tickle his side (belly button height) after laying him on his back. He will move his arms and legs all around. Most night urination or asthma will be cured in a month.

After giving him a bath, tickling the infant on his side will be the best exercise. This exercise causes the body's muscles to move, and any deformity will be balanced out unconsciously.

The most important thing for infants is: Don't give any sugar or sugar products. Sugar will cause an acidic condition after removing calcium from the body. Most children's sicknesses will be cured simply by stopping sugar or sugar products.

Baby care. Our life starts in mother's womb. Therefore, the wellbeing of pregnant mothers—breathing, diet, motion (activities), and thinking—is most important for the good health of the baby.

Give a bath every day after the baby is born. Crying is baby's exercise. Therefore, don't give milk right after the baby cries. The baby goes to sleep after crying awhile and then cries again, louder than before. At this time give milk. Because he had a good exercise (crying), he drinks very well. If such training is given during baby time, the baby will grow up with strong endurance.

For the milk, mother's milk is best. I often see babies whose faces are deformed because they are drinking milk from a bottle. Why has this happened? If a baby drinks from mother's breast, mother changes holding the baby from left to right side and vice versa. However, when bottle feeding, mother always holds the baby in the left hand and gives the bottle with the right hand. Therefore, the baby is always facing one way. This is the reason that the baby's face will be deformed.

Also, it is said that a baby grown by mother's milk is 4 times stronger than a baby grown with cow's milk.

Baby's clothes should not be too tight, so that the baby can move freely. The reason for this is so they can automatically correct any possible deformations. Also, let them be naked once a day so they can move the body very freely.

When weaning from milk, the mother should give the baby whole foods after masticating them well in her mouth. If mother does not have enough milk, she should eat dandelion, which will increase milk production. When I was jailed in Siberia after World War II, I cultivated dandelion in the backyard and ate the leaves, roots, and flowers; this made up for my shortage of greens (lack of vitamins).

Part 2

Basic Sotai Exercises

In all exercises: When body is moving, exhale slowly. When movement stops, inhale quickly. Then exhale again slowly.

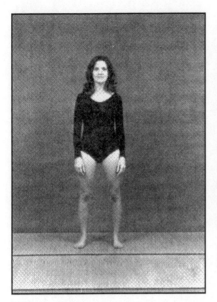 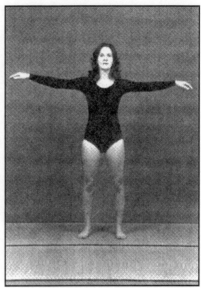

1. Stand with feet straight forward and legs apart at width of hips, backbone and hip straight, and eyes focused straight ahead. Raise arms straight out to sides, exhaling. Holding arms out, inhale quickly. Hold breath three seconds, then exhale quickly; at the same time, let arms drop quickly down to position at side of body. Do this 3 to 5 times.

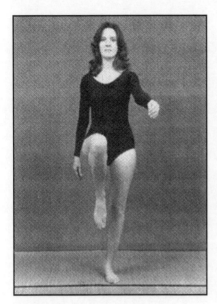 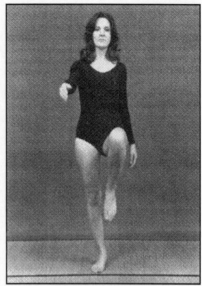

2. Stand with feet together, raise one leg so knee is straight, foot pointing forward, not down. At the same time, raise opposite arm out to shoulder level in front of body. Other arm should swing backward. Put foot down forcefully, raise other leg and repeat in marching fashion, 30 to 50 times.

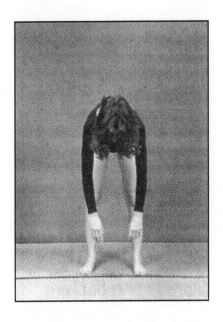

3. With feet apart (width of hips) and arms relaxed, slowly bend forward from the waist letting the arms move toward touching the ground. Exhale while bending. While in this bent position, raise head and inhale quickly.

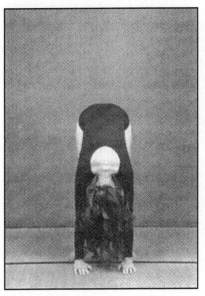

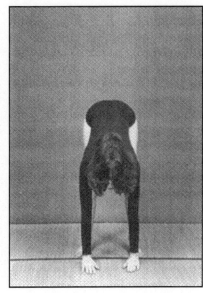

Exhale slowly, move to upright position. Continue bending backward as far as possible without using force, placing hands on back of hips for support. Let head drop back, inhale quickly. Exhale again while returning to original upright position. Do this 3 to 5 times.

If it is difficult to bend forward very far, before bending forward place hands on hips and move hips to the right and left, forward and backward.

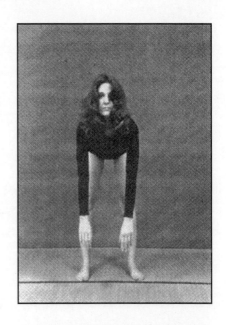

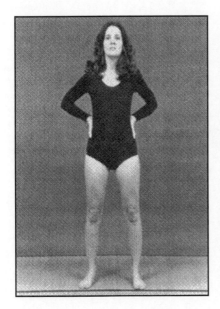

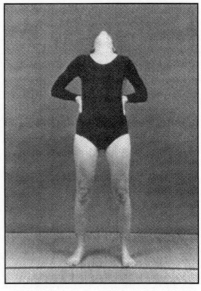

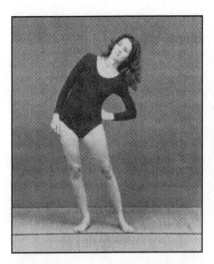 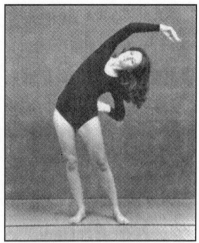

4. Standing with feet apart (width of hips), place left hand on left hip and move right hip outward. Exhaling slowly, raise right arm extended up in an arc over your head and bend body toward the left. Inhale quickly at the end of motion. Then exhale slowly while moving arm slowly back to side.

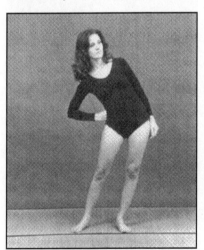 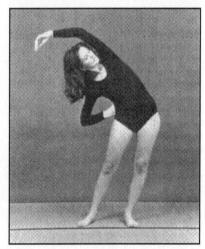

Repeat on opposite side. Repeat 3 to 5 times. Then determine which side has greater ease of movement. Repeat 2 more on easy side and finish by one more time on the side that has more stress.

5. Feet apart (width of hips), arms extended out to sides at shoulder height, relaxed. Left foot remains on the ground, raise right heel off the ground as you slowly turn the body towards the left as far as possible without forcing. (Right arm moves out in front, left arm back.) Exhale slowly while turning. Then inhale quickly and turn to face front again. Do on other side. Repeat 3 to 5 times. Try doing it a couple more times on the side with less stress and finish with one more time on the difficult side.

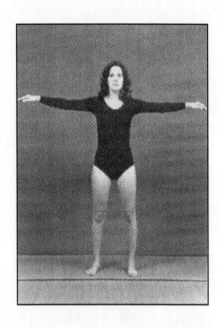

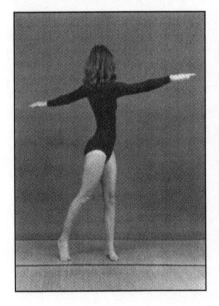

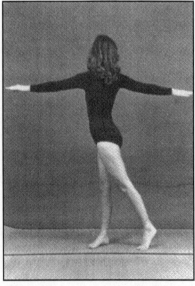

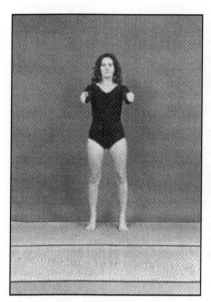 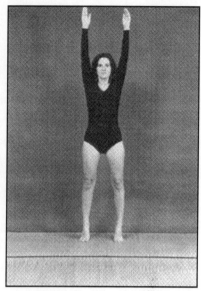

6. With feet apart, raise arms up in front of the body, lifting both heels off the ground until you are standing on toes. Quickly inhale. Hold breath three seconds, then quickly exhale and drop and release arms and heels down to original position. Repeat 3 to 5 times. For one who has difficulty in stretching out, try to move the body weight to the left or right slightly and then stretch out.

7. Stand with arms extended and hands against a wall or hanging onto a support bar, feet apart, with weight on both sides. Bend knees as far down as possible. Exhale slowly, move hips right and left a little bit. Repeat 3 to 5 times. Repeat 2 times on the side with more ease. Then finish with once on difficult side.

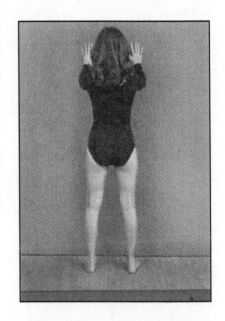

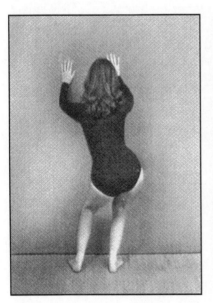

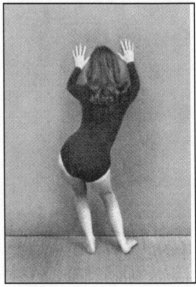

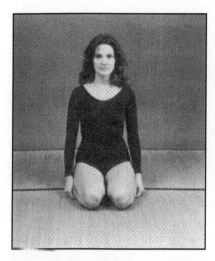 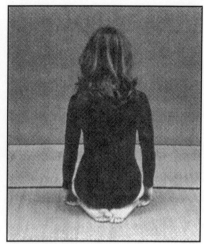

8. Sit on the floor, back straight (in cross-legged position or with feet underneath bottom—seiza). For right handed persons, right toe over the left toe. For left handed persons, vice versa. Men, knees apart 2 palm width; women, knees apart 1 palm width.

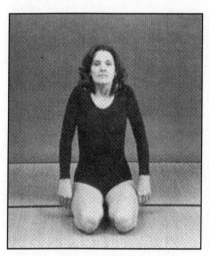 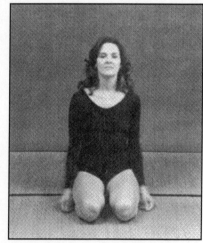

Exhaling slowly, raise shoulders up toward ears. Inhale quickly, hold breath 3 seconds then release (drop shoulders) and exhale quickly. Repeat 3 to 5 times.

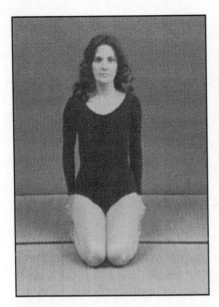 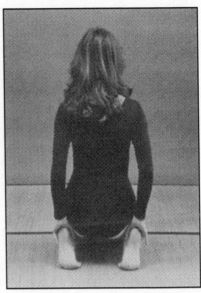

9. Sit with knees together, feet apart, raised up on toes underneath bottom. Place hands on heels. Exhaling, slowly bend forward and move waist in a circle at a 45-degree angle. At top or bottom of circle, inhale quickly like a top slowing down. Then continue exhaling slowly. Five times clockwise, then 5 times counterclockwise.

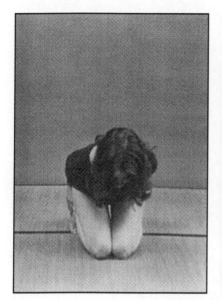
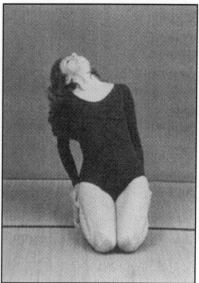

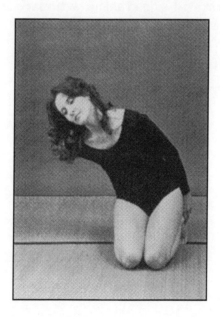

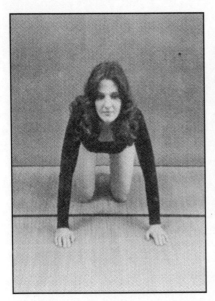 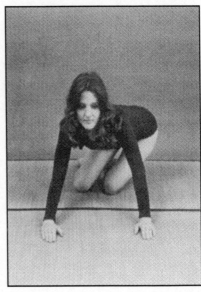

10. In a position like a 4-legged animal with hands on the floor, move hips left to right, then shoulders left to right. Then move body forward and backward. Repeat 5 times.

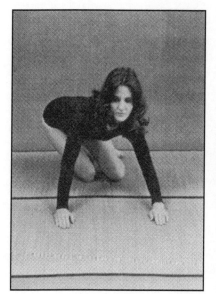
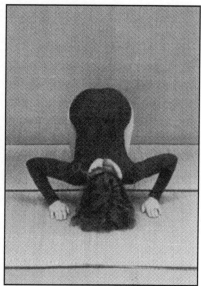

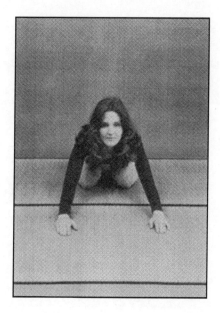

11. Lie on stomach, hands placed under head. Turn head to left, move left knee up toward head as far as possible without forcing. Inhale and return leg to outstretched position.

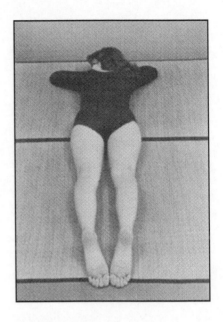

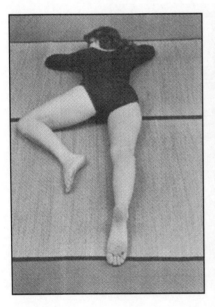

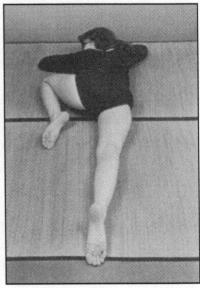

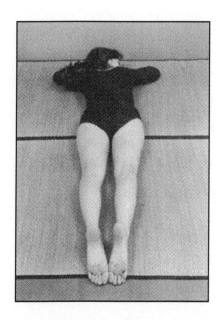

Turn head to right side and re-peat, moving right leg. Repeat 3 to 5 times. Do 2 more times on easy side; then once on dif-ficult side to finish.

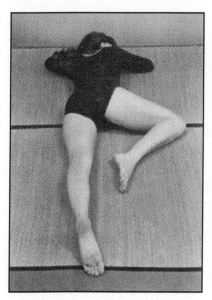

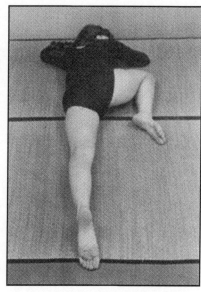

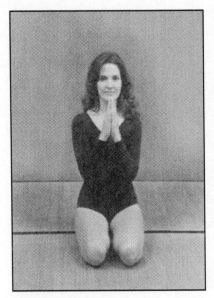 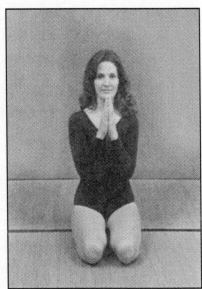

12. Sit on the floor, back straight. Clap hands hard 20 times.

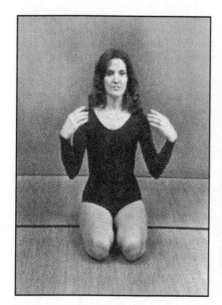 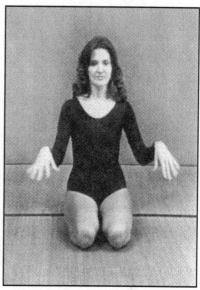

13. Sit on the floor, back straight. Shake hands vigorously 15 times.

Part 3

Basic Sotai Exercises with Helper

Sotai means moving the body to correct imbalance in muscles and joints, which is the beginning of sickness or part of sickness. The movement should never be forced (too hard). After these exercises, you should feel comfortable and balanced.

For these exercises, 2 persons are involved: **A**, being treated, and **B**, applying the treatment.

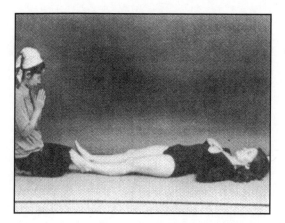

14. A lies in a relaxed position on his back with legs outstretched and hands on chest.

B lifts **A**'s feet by pulling each set of toes, shaking gently,

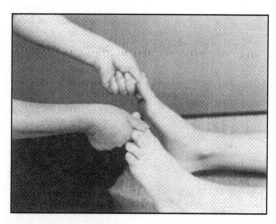

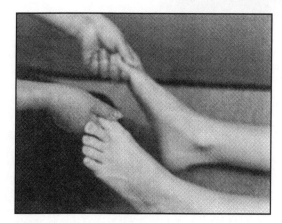

and ending with the big toe.

B should place thumbs on **A**'s ankles (center, inside).

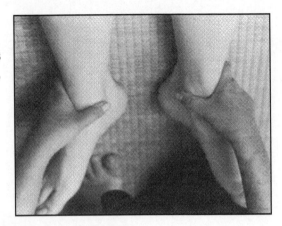

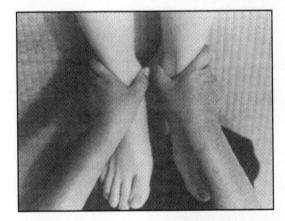

Determine (from position of thumbs) which leg is longer.

Place **A**'s longer leg against **B**'s knee.

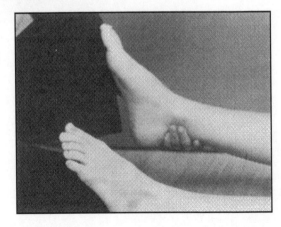

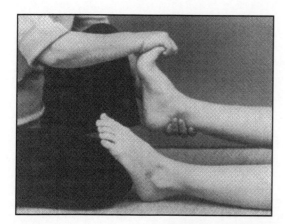

B places one hand underneath the foot of **A**'s shorter leg on the Achilles tendon.

B flexes **A**'s foot back and forth with the other hand and also occasionally pulls the leg with the hand underneath.

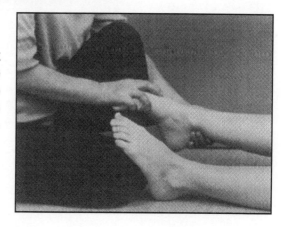

15. After doing this treatment, sore hips or a dull and tired body will be about half cured. Person being treated should lie on the back in a relaxed position with hands on chest and knees up.

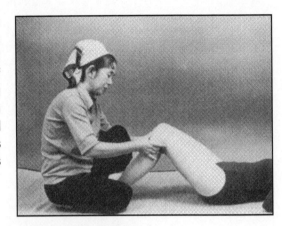

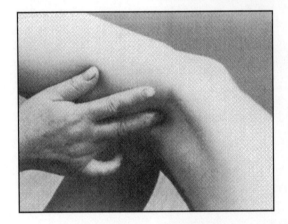

Partner should find the point on the back of the knee where pressure causes pain and ask which knee has more pain.

Sitting in a kneeling position facing the leg with most pain, **B** holds one hand over the top of **A**'s foot and the other hand on top of **A**'s knee.

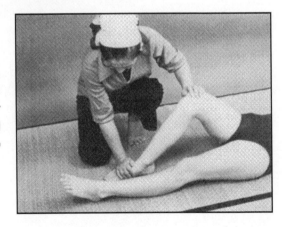

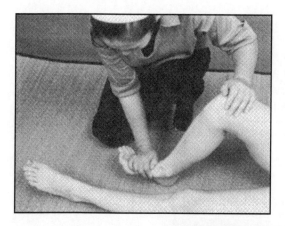

B should begin by instructing **A** to exhale slowly and raise his toes up off the ground (keeping heel down). **B** should press down on **A**'s foot as **A** tries to raise it.

B instructs **A** to inhale quickly. Hold breath 3 seconds, then exhale quickly, relaxing foot. **B** releases pressure as **A** quickly exhales.

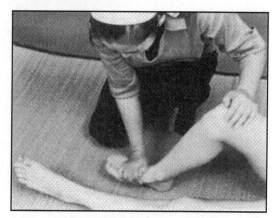

This quick release at the end causes the release of tension and will alleviate pain. In order for the actions of **A** and **B** to be coordinated, **B** should tell when to raise foot, when to inhale, and when to release. After repeating 4 times on first leg, **B** should check back of the knee again to see if the pain has lessened. Touch finger to the back of the knee that didn't receive treatment and then check the other side. All checking procedures after treatment should be like this. First check the side that didn't receive treatment and then check the side on which treatment was given.

16. For relief of back and hip pain, **A** lies in same position as for previous treatment. **B** moves **A**'s knees to both the left and right sides to touch the floor and to determine which side is more difficult. **A** should lean knees toward difficult side.

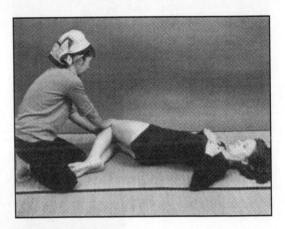

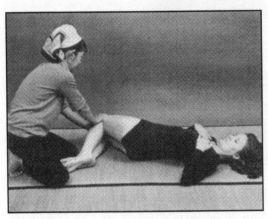

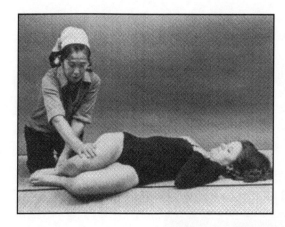

As before, **B** should instruct **A** when to exhale and move legs, when to inhale, and when to release.

B places hands on **A**'s knees and applies resistance as **A** tries to raise knees up toward center position.

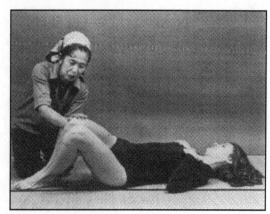

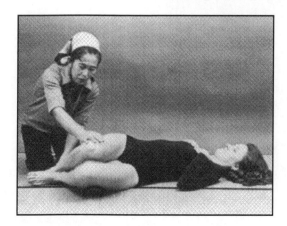

17. For sore hips, **A** lies in the same position and **B** moves **A**'s legs up toward **A**'s chest one at a time to determine which side is more difficult. On the side which is more difficult, **B** sits against **A**'s feet and places **A**'s foot on **B**'s knee, holding both hands on the middle of **A**'s foot. **A** should exhale slowly and raise hips off the ground as **B** applies pressure downward on **A**'s knee, then inhale, hold breath for 3 seconds and release.

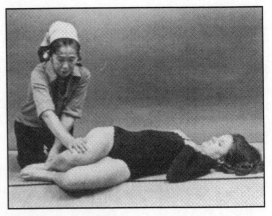

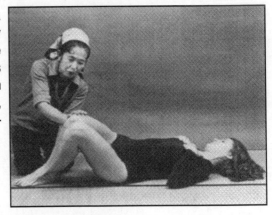

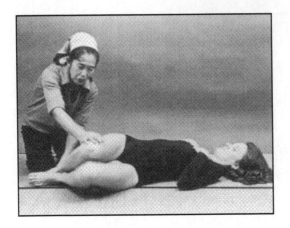

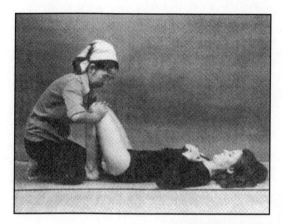

18. Same position. **B** sits facing **A** and with his hands on both sides of **A**'s knees applies pressure inward as **A** tries to separate and move knees outward.

Then raise hips up off ground, inhale quickly, hold breath for 3 seconds, and release. Repeat 4 times.

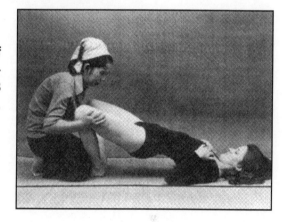

19. A lies on her back with arms down along sides. **B** pulls **A**'s arms to see which side has most resistance from the shoulder.

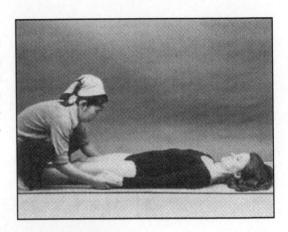

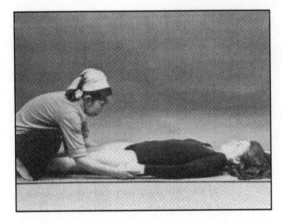

On the side with most resistance, **B** pulls down on the back arm while **A** raises shoulder up toward the head, exhaling slowly, then inhaling quickly. Hold the breath for 3 seconds, exhale, and release. Repeat 3 times. Check.

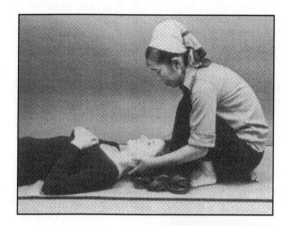

20. For neck pain, ringing in the ears, headache, dizziness (trouble from the neck up: eye, nose, teeth, etc.). **A** lies on her back.

B places her hands on the back of **A**'s neck and applies pressure on either side to determine which side has more pain.

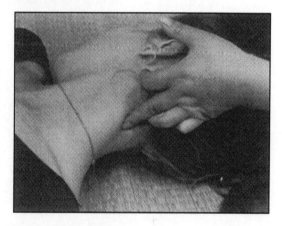

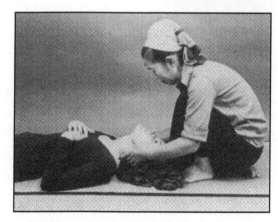

Then placing the middle finger of each hand under the neck and thumbs alongside chin, **B** should instruct **A** to exhale slowly and raise chin up until the top of the head touches the floor.

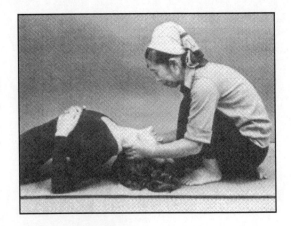

Then raise breast up.

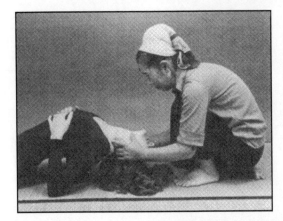

A should then inhale quickly and hold it for a couple of seconds, exhale and release.

When **A** releases, **B** should turn **A**'s head toward the difficult side and slightly pull head up away from the body. Repeat 3 times. Check.

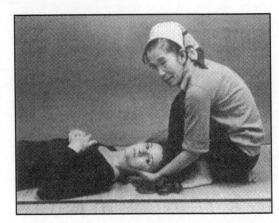

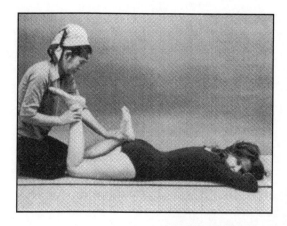

21. For back pain or hip pain, if hands cannot touch the ground when bending from the waist, then too much animal products have been eaten.

A lies on her stomach, **B** bends **A**'s legs from knee so that the heel touches the buttocks.

On the side with most difficulty, **B** holds **A**'s ankle with leg and heel touching bottom (or close if it is not possible to touch).

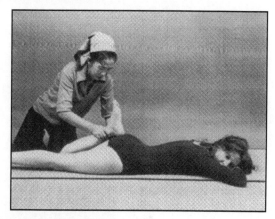

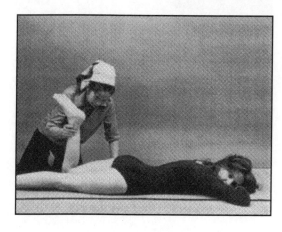

B should apply resistance as **A** moves leg to outstretched position (exhale).

Then raise knee off the ground about 3 inches (not any higher than this or kneecaps will be broken), inhale quickly, hold breath for 3 seconds, then release. Repeat 5 times. Check.

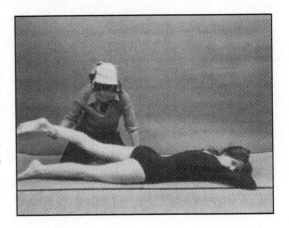

22. For hip pain and for correcting the alignment of the spine.

A lies on her stomach. She moves each leg one at a time, bending the knees along the floor up toward head, and turns her head toward whichever leg is moving. Determine which side is more difficult.

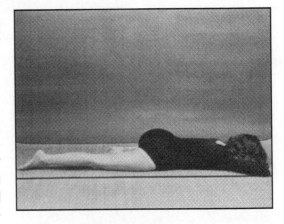

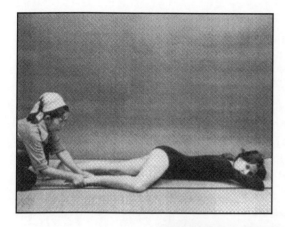

On the more difficult side, **B** holds onto **A**'s ankles and applies resistance as **A** moves leg up to the point where the heel reaches to the knee of the other leg.

Then **A** inhales quickly and holds for 3 seconds and then releases.

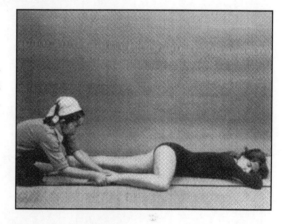

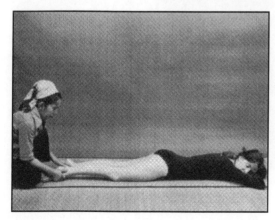

Upon release, **B** should pull **A**'s leg back to outstretched position. Repeat 5 times. Check, **B** holding both of **A**'s feet.

23. This exercise is good for female reproductive and urinary organs. **A** lies on stomach with feet together up in the air and knees bent. **B** places right hand on Achilles tendon and left hand underneath the toe part of the feet and moves the feet toward the left. Then **B** switches the hand position and moves the feet toward the right. On the most difficult side, **B** applies resistance as **A** moves feet toward center position from position pointing either left or right. Repeat 5 times.

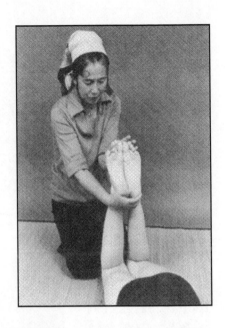

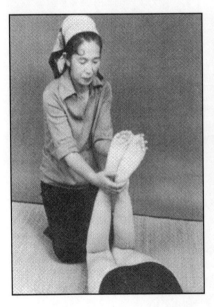

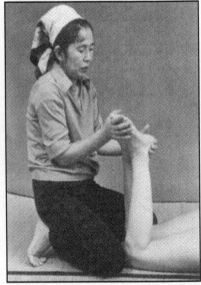

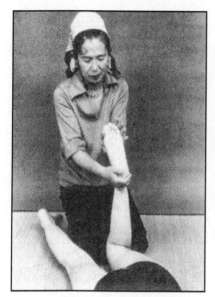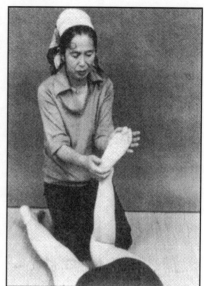

Then moving each foot individually in like manner, determine the
difficult direction and repeat 5 times for each foot. Check at the end
to see if movement has become easier.

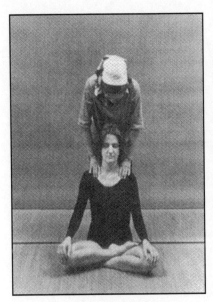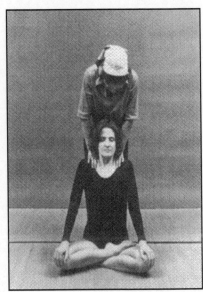

24. This exercise is for shoulder ache, feeling like weight on shoulders is too much, pressure on shoulders, heavy feeling, or tightness in the shoulders. **A** in sitting position, **B** stands behind **A** with one hand on either shoulder. **B** should press down first on the right shoulder then the left shoulder to see which side moves with the greatest difficulty. On the difficult side, **B** presses down on the shoulder while **A** raises the shoulder up, exhaling, then **A** inhales quickly and holds for 3 seconds and releases. Repeat 5 times. Check.

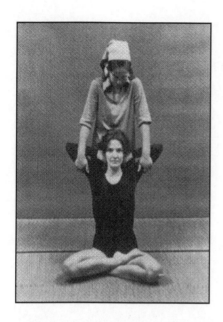

25. A in a sitting position with hands locked behind the neck, **B** stands behind **A** with the knees touching **A**'s back, holding onto **A**'s elbows. She turns **A**'s body to the left and right to see which side moves with more difficulty. On the difficult side, **B** applies resistance as **A** (starting at turned position) moves body toward original position. Exhale and inhale, hold breath 3 seconds, and release. Repeat 5 times. Check.

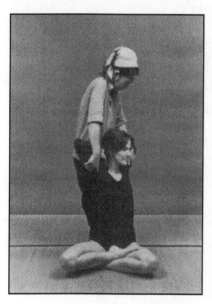

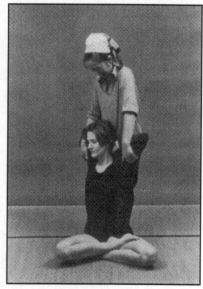

26. This exercise is good for shoulder or arm ache. **A** sits and stretches out left arm. On left side **B** faces opposite direction of **A** and holds left hand on **A**'s shoulder. **B**'s right hand holds **A**'s hand. **B** twists **A**'s hand in front and back to see which side is more difficult. On the difficult side, **B** applies pressure as **A** turns hand from twisted direction in towards center. Repeat 4 times. Check. Repeat the entire treatment on other arm. Release should be of the whole arm including the shoulder. Check the easy side first then the difficult side.

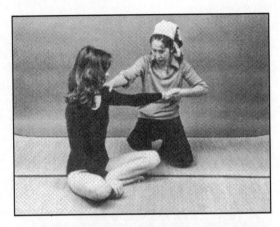

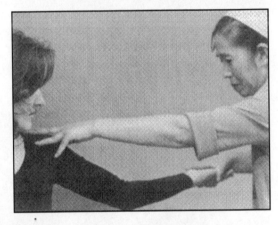

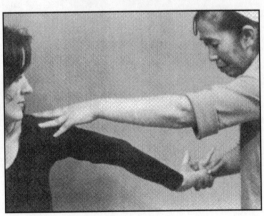

Part 4

Sotai Treatment According to Illness

27. Headache and to straighten the neck section of the spine.

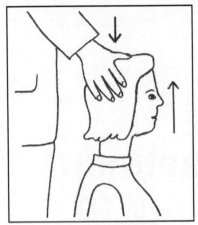

A is in a sitting position (on the floor or in a chair). B places both thumbs on the crown of A's head with other fingers down the sides of the head. B pushes down with the thumbs as A pushes up, exhaling slowly; then inhale quickly and hold for a couple of seconds, then release. Repeat 5 times.

28. Headache on side of the head. Generally, right-handed people will have headaches on the left side because the left side is contracted and the neck (cervical) vertebrae will be out of alignment.

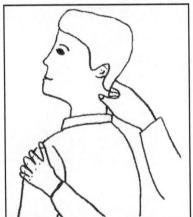 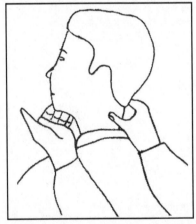

B applies pressure on both sides of the back of A's neck to see which side has the most pain. If pain is on the left side, B should place right hand on back of A's neck (thumb to the left side, fingers to the right side) and place his left hand around A's chin, turning A's head to the left. From this turned position, B should apply resistance as A tries to turn his head toward center. Exhale slowly while turning, then inhale quickly, then release. Repeat 5 times. Check.

29. Dizziness from unbalanced body. Dizziness can be from many causes, but one cause may be scoliosis (crooked spine).

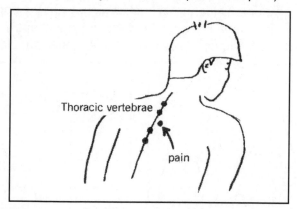

To find the problem area of the spine, **B** pushes on points one inch to the right side and one inch to the left side of the third thoracic vertebra to find which point is more painful. If the person is right-handed, the right side will likely be most painful because the vertebra will be moved over to the right. If pain is on the right side, treatment should be as follows:

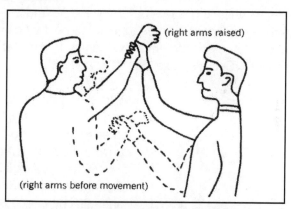

A is in a sitting position with right elbow tight against the body and hand raised up. **B** kneels facing **A**, right hand grasping **A**'s right wrist. **B** then applies resistance as **A** (exhaling) raises arm up and slightly out to the right side. When arm is raised, **A** inhales quickly and holds for 3 seconds, then releases. Repeat 5 times. Check points on back to see if pain is reduced.

30. More for dizziness and/or scoliosis.

A lies on stomach, relaxed, with arms down to sides. **B** sees whether the right side or left side of **A**'s back is higher. On the opposite side from the higher side, **B** should hold **A**'s ankle and apply resistance as **A** tries to bring knee up toward head (**A**'s head should be turned

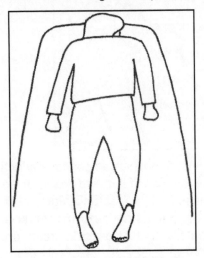 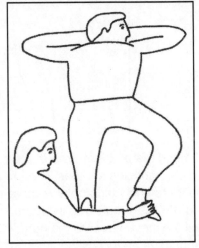

to face side on which leg is raising). Hold awhile and then relax with quick exhalation. Repeat 5 times, check to see if sides of back are now even, and check points on both sides of third vertebra to see if pain is reduced. (See also exercise 22, page 88.)

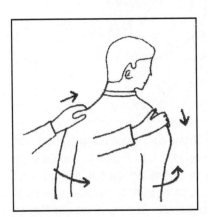

A in sitting position, **B** kneeling or sitting behind **A** with one hand on each of **A**'s shoulders, should turn **A**'s body to left and right to find the most difficult direction. **B** should turn **A**'s body toward the most difficult direction and apply resistance as **A** tries to twist to center, exhaling slowly. When **A** is at center, he inhales quickly, holding 3 seconds, then releases. Repeat five times and check.

31. Insomnia.

When people have insomnia, the back of the neck is very rigid.

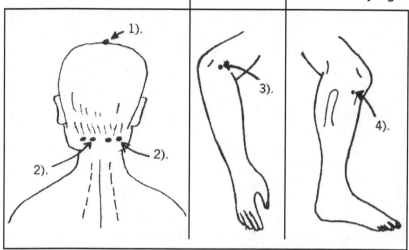

Points to treat: 1). Locate on top of the head the intersection of a line running between the ears. With the thumbs, press 5 times. 2). On back of neck at bottom edge of skull bone about 1 inch out

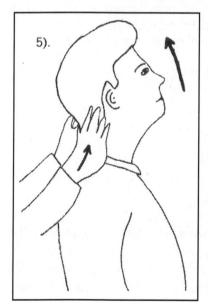

from center, apply pressure with thumb and second finger, pushing up while supporting head by holding other hand on forehead. Repeat 3 times. 3). With arm bent slightly, find point just outside of wrinkle on inside of elbow. Apply pressure 5 times to each arm. 4). On leg 1-1/2" out from bone sticking out below kneecap (this point is located in a slight indentation), apply pressure five times on each leg. 5). **A** in sitting position with head bent forward, **B** holds hands on back of **A**'s neck and applies resistance pressure as **A** tries to lift chin up and head back. Repeat 5 times.

32. Stiff neck. If this happens in the morning after waking up, it probably comes from sitting in one position for a long time like watching TV.

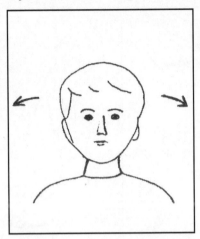 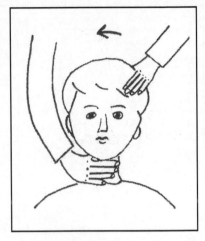

a). **A** in sitting position, **B** standing or kneeling behind **A**. **B** moves **A**'s head to either side, tipping head down—not turning. On most difficult side, **B** places one hand on **A**'s chin and one hand on the side of **A**'s head toward crown and applies resistance as **A** moves head in one direction as far as comfortably possible, exhaling. **A** inhales quickly then releases. Repeat 3 times. Check.

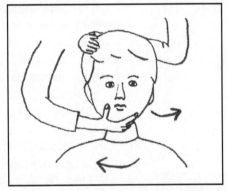

b). **A** in sitting position; **B** places one hand on **A**'s chin and one hand on the side of **A**'s head and moves head to either side, rotating chin. On most difficult side, **B** applies resistance as **A** turns head. Then **A** releases suddenly as in the other treatments. Repeat 3 times. Check.

33. Shoulder Ache. If person is over 50, shoulder ache is caused by contraction in legs. First, you should do sotai treatments for legs, then this one for shoulders.

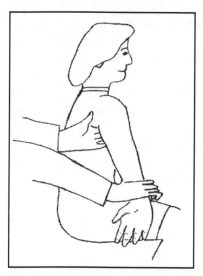

A sitting, **B,** standing behind **A**, places hands on **A**'s shoulders and pushes down as **A** lifts shoulders up. Stop, deeply inhale, and quickly relax by exhaling. Repeat 5 times. (See also exercise 24, page 92.)

34. Difficulty of arm movement.

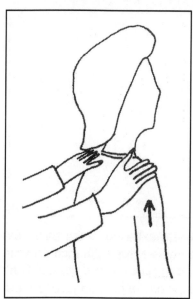

A in sitting position, **B** presses point on back 1-1/2" above **A**'s armpit. On the side with most pain, **A** holds arm out to side and turns wrist, rotating front or back, to find which direction is most difficult. **B** holds **A**'s wrist and places other hand on **A**'s shoulder, turns wrist in direction of most difficulty and applies pressure as **A** tries to turn wrist toward center. Repeat 5 times. Check point on back to see if pain is reduced.

For pain in the shoulder joint (which is difficult to get rid of), always do sotai treatments for legs first, then do this treatment for the shoulder joint.

35. For difficulty moving arms up straight.

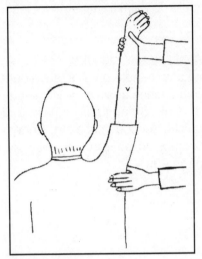

A should raise each arm straight up from shoulder to determine which arm moves with most difficulty and pain. On difficult side, **B** holds **A**'s wrist with one hand and places other hand on back at **A**'s armpit. **B** holds arm up with elbow bent 90 degrees and applies resistance as **A** moves arm down to side. Repeat 5 times; check by raising easy arm, then difficult arm.

36. Hip pain. If pain is so great that you cannot move at all, better to see a doctor.

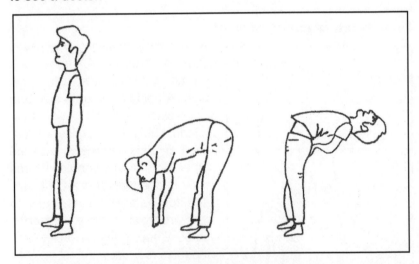

a). Stand naturally. Bend body forward, exhaling. Then back, exhaling. Determine which direction is easier. Repeat bending to the easier direction 5 times. Then slowly bend once in the more difficult direction. If there is still pain, bend to the easier direction 5 or 6 more times.

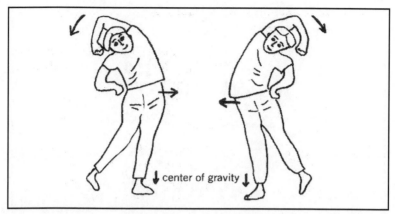

b). Stand naturally. With weight on right leg, raise right arm curved up over head and bend body to left side, exhaling, weight on right side; left heel up. Try on both sides to see which side is more difficult. Repeat on easy side 5-6 times. Then check to see if pain is gone on difficult side. If pain is still there, repeat slowly again 5-6 times on easy side. Check again on difficult side.

37. More on hip pain.

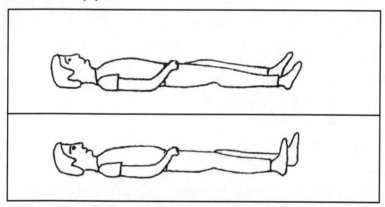

a). People with pain in hips usually have legs of different length. Lie on back. With toes pointing up, stretch each heel forward to see which leg has pain. On easy side, repeat stretching 5-6 times, exhaling slowly. Check difficult side to see if pain is reduced. Repeat again on easy side 5-6 times. Check again.

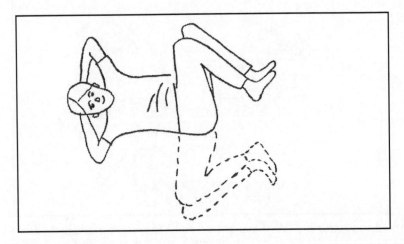

b). Lie on back with knees up and together, feet together and hands behind head. Move knees together to touch floor on either side. On easy side, repeat 5-6 times, exhaling slowly. Check difficult side. Repeat 5-6 times on easy side again. Check difficult side.

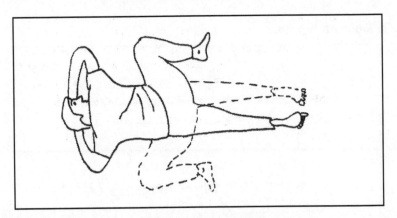

c). Lie on stomach with hands beneath head. Turn head to right side and move right knee up toward head. Turn head to left side and move left knee up toward head. Repeat 5-6 times on easy side only. Check difficult side. If still difficult, repeat again 5-6 times on easy side. Check again.

38. Stiffness. Older people often have difficulty moving after waking up.

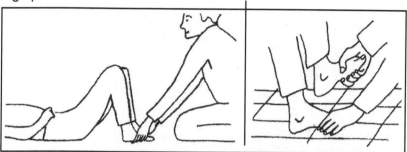

a). **A** lies on back with hands on chest and knees bent, feet flat on floor. **B** presses on a point at back of kneecap on each leg to see which side has more pain. On side with most pain, **B** places his hand on top of **A**'s foot and applies resistance as **A** raises toe up as far as possible, exhaling slowly. Then **A** inhales quickly, holds a couple of seconds, and releases. Repeat 5 times and check points on back of knees again. b). **A** lies on back, knees up, hands on chest. **B** finds

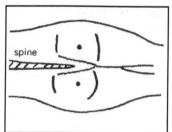

point on buttocks halfway between tip of spine and hip bones. Apply thumb pressure on either side to see which side has most pain. On side with most pain, **B** moves **A**'s knees together over to one side, touching floor. **B** applies resistance as **A** raises knees up toward center; exhale, inhale, and release. Repeat 5 times, then check points again. When pain is gone, then body can move. (See also exercise 16, page 80.)

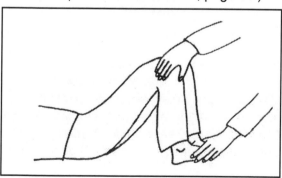

39. Stomach pain. Pain may be caused by gas trapped in folds of large intestines.

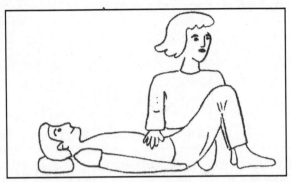

A lies on back with knees up (to relax stomach). **B** places hand flat on **A**'s stomach and pushes as **A** exhales slowly. Repeat 7 times, waiting a bit between each repeat to allow gas to move through intestines.

40. Sharp stomachache.

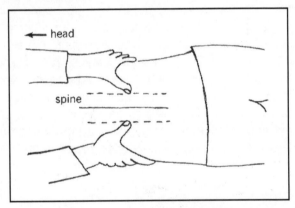

A lies on stomach, hands under head. **B** presses hard with both thumbs on points on either side of spine about 1 inch up from the lowest rib. Press the point that causes the most pain. **A** will probably hold in breath because of pain and may squirm to try and escape pain, but **B** should keep pressing until **A** starts breathing normally. **A** will start breathing normally when pain is gone so **B** can then discontinue pressing.

41. Expanded stomach (uneasy or bloated feeling—acid or upset).

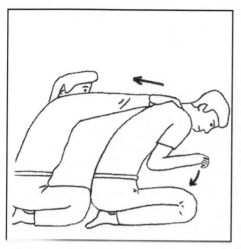

A sits with feet under buttocks, holding elbows in tight to sides and hands out front. **A** pulls in stomach and bends forward with back rounded. **B** sits behind **A** with knees against back of **A**'s hips and holds onto **A**'s shoulders and applies resistance. **A** bends forward while exhaling then inhaling quickly; hold a couple of seconds and release quickly (exhale). Repeat several times.

42. Stomach out of position or chronic women's disease. Repeated every day will help prevent miscarriage. Right-handed people will have contracted muscle on back of hip on left side, opposite for left-handed people.

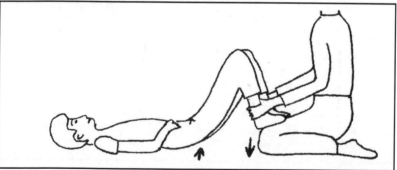

A lies on back with hands on chest or stomach and knees up. **B** sits facing **A** and puts **A**'s feet on top of **B**'s thighs. **A** should raise hips off floor and move one foot in marching fashion (right-handed person, press down left foot; left-handed, press down right foot). **A** should exhale slowly and inhale quickly about every 3-5 times he presses foot. After 4 exhales, **A** should release and drop hips to floor. Repeat 5 times.

43. Pain in legs (from walking, climbing mountains, or farm work).

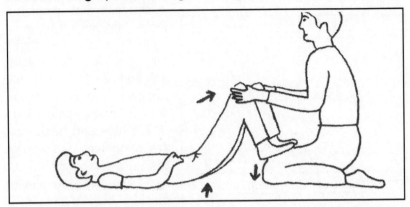

a). **A** lies on back with knees up. **B** sits facing **A** with **A**'s feet on top of **B**'s thighs. **B** places hands on **A**'s knees and applies resistance inward. **A** raises hips and knees, exhaling; then inhales quickly, holding 3 seconds, then releases and drops hips to floor. Repeat 5 times.

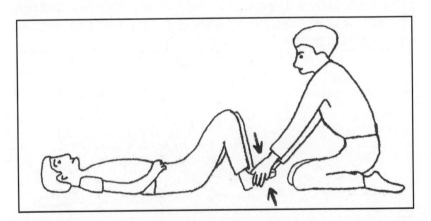

b). **A** lies on back with knees up, feet flat on floor. **B** sits at **A**'s feet and puts hands on top of **A**'s feet, applying resistance as **A** lifts toes and raises them up toward front part of leg. **A** should inhale, hold and release (exhale) quickly.

44. Dull, heavy feeling in legs (during the summer months).

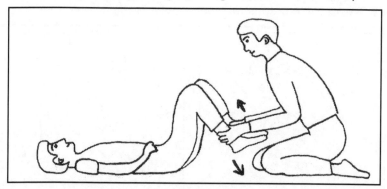

A lies on back with knees up, and **B** sits facing **A** with **A**'s feet over **B**'s thighs (but not touching). **B** holds **A**'s ankles and applies resistance in direction toward **A** (push up) as **A** puts each foot down alternately in marching fashion 7 times. Then **A** should stand up and march to see how legs now feel lighter.

45. Knee pain. This exercise is for the person who finds it difficult to sit in seiza position because of pain in knees (not for pain in knees caused by infection).

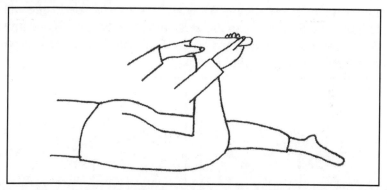

A lies on stomach, one foot up in the air at 90-degree angle; **B** turns **A**'s foot in each direction to see which side is most difficult. On most difficult side, **B** holds **A**'s foot over to side and applies resistance as **A** rotates foot toward center. **A** should inhale, hold, then quickly relax. Repeat 5 times on one foot. Check, then repeat 5 times on other foot and check. If pain is gone, **A** will be able to sit in seiza position.

46. Twisted wrist or ankle. Always move from painful side to easy side. Never force on painful side.

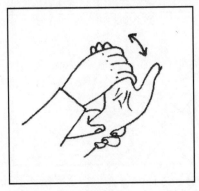 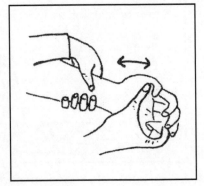

A holds arm out with back of hand up. **B** holds one hand on **A**'s wrist and the other hand around **A**'s fingers, and moves **A**'s hand both up and down, bending at wrist to see which is the side with pain. Then starting at painful side, **B** applies resistance as **A** moves hand toward easy side. **A** should inhale, hold breath, and release quickly. Repeat 5 times.

Next, **A** holds palm up. **B** places one hand around **A**'s palm and one hand on **A**'s wrist and moves **A**'s wrist from side to side to see which side has pain. Starting from the side with pain, **B** applies resistance as **A** moves hand toward easy side. **A** should inhale, hold breath, and release quickly. Repeat 5 times.

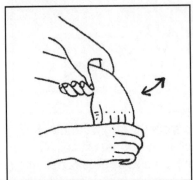 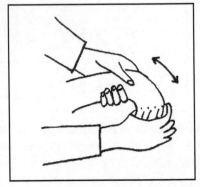

Next treatment is repeated as above but with palm down rather than up. Repeat 5 times.

47. Bed-wetting and child asthma. Continue treatment every day for one or two months. Can cure if asthma or bed-wafting is not very serious, and if not feeding any meat or sugar.

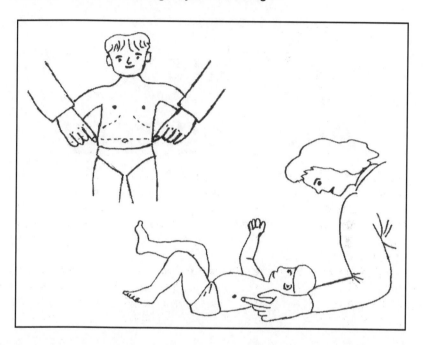

With baby lying on back, **B** should lightly tickle points on both sides in line with belly button. The baby will move all around and the activity will strengthen internal organs and straighten the spine. Continue for a couple of minutes.

Part 5

Autobiography

Fifty Years in the Medical Professional

Symptomatic cure is the lowest medicine. I will be 80 years old next year. My wife of 56 years died a few years ago. I am sorry. I married her when I was still a student in Niigata Medical College. My eldest son was born when I was drafted. After I was released from the army, I continued the study of neurology at Tohoku Imperial University, under the guidance of Professor Toshihiko Fujita. I spent my days studying whatever I wanted to study. They were happy days.

Of course, my income was small. My house had a bathtub but no money to heat up the water. So my wife went to her parents' home to take a bath with her baby. My wage was 75 yen per month and the rent was 20 yen. I often sold my used books whenever I needed money. Renting out my wife's bridal costume brought us unexpected money. I could afford to buy only one plastic goldfish toy for my eldest son. I went to school with a lunchbox; I never ate at the soba restaurant even though soba was my favorite food.

When I received some extra salary, I bought my wife a kimono sash. I still remember how much she enjoyed it. However, I didn't want to make her life harder, so I decided to work at a clinic that was located in Hakodate City, in Hokkaido. It was 5 years after my graduation from medical school.

School Health Administration. My job at the clinic was to give treatment to the sick, in which I had no experience. Although I didn't have experience, I worked hard. However, the owner of this clinic disappeared in my third month on this job. The clinic was closed and

I lost the job.

Then the head of the City Hospital arranged a job for me—a health administrator for over 20 of the city's elementary schools.

During that time, I studied children's dental sickness and concluded that sugar and sugary foods are the cause of dental decay. Brushing teeth does not much help if one eats sugar and sugary candy.

After working at this job for 2 years, I quit so that I could help my friend who had just started the nonprofit Hakodate Hospital and who could not get enough help.

Not satisfied with orthodox Western medicine, I searched Oriental medicine. I worked in this hospital for 5 years. I treated injuries as well as sicknesses of the internal organs. I encountered all kinds of sicknesses. I had question after question. Medical books couldn't give me answers. Many patients left me and went to practitioners of Oriental medicine. They seemed to be satisfied with the treatments of Oriental medicine. Therefore, I wanted to know more about Oriental medicine.

To me, surgical patients were the most difficult to handle. So when I had such patients, I asked a honetsugishi (Japanese chiropractor) to treat them. I watched his treatments and learned his techniques. I invited masseurs, acupuncturists, moxa-therapists, etc. They were all eager to teach me their techniques.

Some of their techniques, I noticed, cure pains by moving the body parts toward the unpainful direction. I realized that sickness has a relationship with bones and muscles.

At that time, a sailor had fallen from a mast and hit his forehead and broken the bone. The bone was concaved. Only surgery can bring out this concaved bone. I pushed several points of the skull. There was a very painful point just opposite the concaved bone. I tried to push this point gently without causing pain. He felt good. I pushed this point every day. Two to three weeks later, the concaved forehead started to come out. I continued pushing, and 2-3 months later, it was almost normal. This fact surprised me because no medical books mentioned this.

Unknown masters of medicine. When I was an elementary school health administrator, I met a man who had a special painless technique for cleaning children's ear wax within a minute, while an ear doctor will take 2-3 days to do so. I asked him the technique. He was more than happy to show me the result of his 50 years of study. He had examined over I million persons and treated more than 120,000. I made a report on his studies in a medical journal.

Later, when I was researching Oriental medicine, there was a master acupuncturist in Hakodate City. He used very thin needles (less than 0.1 mm diameter). He cured pain miraculously without causing any pain upon insertion. I asked him to teach me his technique. However, I couldn't insert such a thin needle. I gave up. About half a year later, I tried it again for my patients. Then I succeeded. Now I can teach this technique in 5 minutes to anyone.

Starting my own clinic in Hakodate City in 1933. I had read a book, *New Studies of Chinese Medicine* by Tadanaho Nakayama (translator's note—this was translated into French by George Ohsawa and was the first acupuncture book in France), that said that Oriental medicine is effective, but the mechanism of the cure cannot be explained in terms of Western medicine. This confirmed my belief that Oriental medicine has something to do with the correction of bones and muscles.

I decided to start my own clinic in 1933 in which I practiced internal medicine as well as surgery. However, I gave herbal medicines to take instead of Western medicines. I studied herbal medicine by reading books written by K. Ohtsuka and K. Yumoto. It was convenient that next door was a pharmacy selling Chinese herbs.

In older times, Oriental doctors concocted medicine to fit the patients. Modern doctors using drugs manufactured by pharmaceutical companies are only relying on their knowledge of pharmacology learned in school.

I began to study sotai treatment. In Chinese medicine, there is herbal medicine and physical medicine. I gave patients this physical medicine or treatment. That is to say, I gave comfortable stimulation on certain acupuncture points. Patients felt better immediately if I gave stimulation in the right place; therefore, I knew right away if I was doing right or not.

Correction should be given to the bones, but bones are connected with muscle and covered with tissue. Therefore, stimulation should be given to the soft tissue that covers the bones.

I found that acupuncture points exist on the skin; however, the degree of pain depends on the stresses on the soft tissues.

Modern Western science diagnoses patients very well chemically, physiologically, and physically. Then they decide to give names for sicknesses. Sometimes they cannot give a name; then the doctor says to his patient, "you are not sick." For doctors, the most difficult problem is when they cannot find any symptoms of sicknesses and yet patients claim uncomfortable feelings.

In such cases, Oriental medicine can handle things better. They use needles, moxa, finger massage, manipulation of bones, etc. To me, all Oriental medicines have the same goal: to correct deformation of body muscle, bones, and tissues.

My clinic in Sendai City. I started writing about my conviction that man is originally healthy, but that sickness starts when the body structure develops deformation. Since learning this while working at Hakodate hospital and my own clinic, I confirmed it again and again and started to write it down. It was the spring of 1937. When I finished writing, I was drafted into the Sino-Japanese War in August. I closed the clinic and went to the front, sending my writings to a magazine, *Chinese Herbs and Medicine.*

I was released and came home in 1940. I started the present clinic at Sendai City in December, 1941.

In order to catch up on newer knowledge, I studied at Tohoku University as a special student. At that time, I cured an acute breathing trouble of one of the professors with acupuncture. I treated patients with acupuncture and sotai mostly because Chinese herbs were difficult to acquire at that time.

Drafted once more. At the end of 1944, I received another notice. This time I went to North Korea. My fifth child was an infant. I thought I may not be able to come back home. However, I could rely on my wife; she would take care of my family. Her character was Fire; she had a strong will to overcome any difficulties.

The War ended in 1945. I was detained in Russia and finally

returned home in 1948. During my detention, a soldier in my camp was a good fortuneteller. He said to me, "Your wife is much stronger than you are. As long as she is at home, your home is safe."

My son graduated from medical school in 1945 and was practicing medicine when I returned home. My wife was well taken care of in my absence; she had cared for five children, a backyard garden, and had rented all the rooms of my clinic to support her finances.

For three years after being back home, I was watching all new developments in modern medicine in Japan. No one mentioned the relationship between the basic structure of the body and medicine. In 1951, I started to write articles for various medical magazines.

Sotai and me at present. I wrote articles on my thoughts on medicine and health for various magazine for over 20 years. There were almost no reactions to my writings. So I stopped writing. Then, one of the agriculture magazines asked me to write some articles in 1974. My articles continued in that magazine for two years.

In 1976, local TV stations interviewed me. Finally NHK (the biggest and only national TV station in Japan) interviewed me and broadcast sotai nationwide. Soon after this, I was asked to give a lecture at Miyagi University at Sendai. Several other universities are asking me to give lectures. My old college friends are showing interest in studying my sotai. If they develop my theory and practice, I will be most happy.

Although my wife never understood or showed interest in my work, she let me do as much as I wanted to do and she watched NHK television with most interest when I was on. A few days after watching this TV program, while eating her favorite kanten dessert from my hand, she suddenly died while her daughter and daughter-in-law were watching her.

Conclusion. During these past 15 years, I learned the basic body structure and the mechanics of body movement. I learned how to apply those movements to medicine. Furthermore, I learned that changes or deformations of the movement systems of the body are related to breathing, eating and drinking, physical movement, and mental activities. Finally, I learned that those 4 activities of man will affect our adaptability to our environment. Therefore, I am learning the antagonism and complementarity between environment, breathing, diet, movement, and thinking.

Perfect health is an ideal state. According to how close we observe the natural law, we will be able to approach such perfect health. However, men have the freedom to live against the natural law. Any actions against the natural law will result in deformations of the body and finally sicknesses. This is cause and effect—the natural law. The correcting of one's activities such as breathing, eating (drinking), movement, and thinking according to the natural law is the highest medicine; the symptomatic cure of sickness, in which I worked solely when I was beginning medicine, is the lowest grade of medicine. This is my conclusion after 50 years in the medical profession.

Our health is like a school report. Some have good grades and some have bad grades. Good or bad depends solely on you. Health science that educates people that health is solely our own responsibility, not that of doctors, is much more needed than symptomatic medicine.

— Keizo Hashimoto, M.D.
Autumn 1976

Other books from the George Ohsawa Macrobiotic Foundation

Acid Alkaline Companion - Carl Ferré; 2009; 111 pp; $15.00
Acid and Alkaline - Herman Aihara; 1986; 121 pp; $9.95
As Easy As 1, 2, 3 - Pamela Henkel and Lee Koch; 1990; 176 pp; $6.95
Basic Macrobiotic Cooking, 20th Anniversary Edition - Julia Ferré; 2007; 288 pp; $17.95
Book of Judo - George Ohsawa; 1990; 150 pp; $14.95
Calendar Cookbook - Cornellia Aihara; 1979; 160 pp; $24.95
Cancer and the Philosophy of the Far East - George Ohsawa; 1981; 165 pp; $14.95
Cooking with Rachel - Rachel Albert; 1989; 328 pp; $12.95
Essential Ohsawa - George Ohsawa, edited by Carl Ferré; 1994; 238 pp; $12.95
French Meadows Cookbook - Julia Ferré; 2008; 135 pp; $17.00
Iron: The Most Toxic Metal - Jym Moon, PhD; 2008; 233 pp; $24.95
Learning from Salmon - Herman Aihara; 1986; 338 pp; $14.95
Macrobiotics: An Invitation to Health and Happiness - George Ohsawa; 1971; 128 pp; $11.95
Naturally Healthy Gourmet - Margaret Lawson with Tom Monte; 1994; 232 pp; $14.95
Philosophy of Oriental Medicine - George Ohsawa; 1991; 153 pp; $7.95
Zen Cookery - G.O.M.F.; 1985; 140 pp; $17.00
Zen Macrobiotics, Unabridged Edition - George Ohsawa, edited by Carl Ferré; 1995; 206 pp; $9.95

A complete selection of macrobiotic books is available from the George Ohsawa Macrobiotic Foundation, P.O. Box 3998, Chico, California 95927; (530) 566-9765. Order toll free: (800) 232-2372.

Printed in Great Britain
by Amazon.co.uk, Ltd.,
Marston Gate.